My Teachers Wear Fur Coats

Lessons From Reiki With Pets

by

Susan Mack and Natalia Krawetz

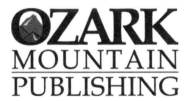

OZARK MOUNTAIN PUBLISHING

PO Box 754
Huntsville, AR 72740
www.ozarkmt.com

For permission, or serialization, condensation, adaptions, or for catalog of other publications, write to: Ozark Mountain Publishing, Inc., PO Box 754, Huntsville, AR 72740, Attn: Permissions Department.

Library of Congress Cataloging-in-Publication Data
Mack, Susan - 1956 -   Krawetz, Natalia - 1949 -
"My Teachers Wear Fur Coats" by Susan Mack and Natalia Krawetz
Lessons learned from Reiki with pets. The Amazing Power of Touch. Using Reiki with pets is a relatively unknown and simple way to: Reduce Pain, Enhance Healing, and Manage Stress.
1. Pets   2. Reiki   3. Touch
I. Mack, Susan, 1956 - II. Krawetz, Natalia, 1949 - III. Title
Library of Congress Catalog Number: 2007928008
ISBN: 978-1-886940-76-5

Cover Art and Layout by www.enki3d.com
Book Design: Julia Degan
Book Set in: Times New Roman, Elephant
Published by

OZARK
MOUNTAIN
PUBLISHING
PO Box 754
Huntsville, AR 72740
www.ozarkmt.com
Printed in The United States of America

For

Reiki Master Friend

and

Lady Cathryn Twinkletoes

Table of Contents

Preface

When I embarked on a career as a professional chef and restaurant owner, I never imagined that a gentle touch therapy called Reiki would change my life. Then in the throes of battling a serious illness, I resorted to touch therapy for my aching arms and hands. I tried massage and physiotherapy, but they were not for me. Someone suggested Reiki.

With Reiki's help, I healed completely. So impressed was I by its effectiveness, that I became a Reiki student. As the healing energy flowed through me, any pets I encountered would come up and shift their bodies into position under my hands. In time, they convinced me to start a pet-oriented practice.

My schooling continued, and I have learned from three of the over two dozen schools of Reiki: Usui Shiki Ryoho, William Lee Rand, and Traditional Japanese Reiki. I've pared my learning from these schools back to the four symbols and accompanying mantras of the modern discoverer of Reiki, Dr. Mikao Usui, because pets have taught me that these are all that I need to use. It is pets who have helped me craft my own approach, so I now practice as an Independent Reiki Master/Teacher unaffiliated with any Reiki school.

Since 1994, I have shared about 2,000 Reiki sessions a year exclusively with pets. Occasionally I share Reiki with their people and can teach them to work with their pets, too. My teachers have largely been cats and dogs; but birds, fish, rabbits, gerbils, turtles, hamsters, guinea pigs, and horses have contributed to my learning as well. In the course of being my instructors, they have run away from me, jumped with pleasure at my arrival, insisted on a play session, bit and scratched my hands, purred deeply, shifted their bodies into position under my hands, filled the room with snores, swatted me when I put my hands where they didn't want them, and vomited, urinated, and defecated on me. They have made sure I pay close attention to get the messages they wish to send.

Soon after I started my work, I took a course on pet wellness taught by Dr. Natalia Krawetz. Natalia has a doctorate in psychology and through career transitions became a holistic health practitioner, a cat behaviorist, and wellness educator. She, too, has been initiated into Reiki (Usui Shiki Ryoho) and is now my student.

When she was a Board member of the Edmonton SPCA, she hired me to work with Sassy, a shelter cat mourning the loss of her long-term, feline companion. As a result, we became well acquainted. We recognized the similarity in our philosophies and the ways in which our skills were complementary. Then we shared several clients - cats and some dogs - Natalia working as a behaviorist and flower essence therapist, and me, as a Reiki practitioner. Over the past ten years we have talked at length about the clients with whom we work, looking at the commonalities across cases, sharing the frustrations, and offering mutual guidance and support.

People told me that I should write a book about my experiences. But my hands work better with pets than they do with the written word - so much so, that Natalia began to edit the column on pet-oriented Reiki that I write. When she retired, she decided that this book should be written. We started with the information in my pet columns, our memories of our detailed conversations throughout the years, her knowledge of holistic health and pets, and her writing skills.

While the bulk of the clients described here are mine, Natalia was deeply involved with one-quarter of them. For the record, she was the one who did Therapeutic Touch with my cat Beakers (described in Chapter Three). All the clients in Chapter Six were initially hers; we continued to keep in close contact to monitor their progress. Before he came to her home, I had worked with Simon (described in Chapter Eight); but once he arrived, she was his prime Reiki person. She played a similar role with Cathryn Twinkletoes (described in Chapter Nine). She is also responsible for formulating the flower remedies described in Appendix C. But rather than weave our voices back and forth between the covers of this book, we decided to speak with one voice: mine.

Before I thank the many pets and people who made this book possible, I want to clarify my use of the term, pet. Some people are comfortable with this term and others are not, because they view it as demeaning. I believe that animals are sentient beings and deserve to be treated with respect and dignity. I chose the term, pet, because it is more commonly known than the alternative, companion animal - even though, I view a pet as a non-human animal who shares regular companionship with a human. As such, a pet can be a friend, a confidant, a helper, a healer, and a teacher.

In the same vein, I have avoided using the term, owner, to describe the human in this relationship. I don't believe pets can be owned. And while I recognize the increasing use of the term, guardian, to mean a legal relationship between the two beings, I prefer the terms caregiver and person - as in, the pet's person, for parity with the phrase, the person's pet.

My deepest thanks go to all the pets and their people who made this book possible: some are composites whose characteristics and stories I melded together into one, some have pseudonyms to protect their people's privacy, but most are identified by their actual names.

I am indebted as well to many members of the Reiki community. Dr. Zoe Thompson and Reiki practitioner, Diane Keno introduced me to Reiki. Reiki Masters Barbara McDaniel, Karen Menshik, Inge Saxena, Wanda Swann, Dr. Marion Taylor, and Lorna Rozak, shared the gift of Reiki as well as guidance and advice. Practitioner Odette Youzwishen gifted the description of Reiki, which is the basis of my brochure and forms much of the first chapter. Practitioner Judy Weir generously shared her information about using Reiki with diabetics. Past editors of the Reiki Practitioners' Association Newsletter, Maja Laird and Val Stewart, assisted with editorial support for my regular column. Thanks also to my Reiki students for continuing to ensure that I communicate the animals' teachings in ways they can understand.

Several veterinary professionals have my gratitude as well: Dr. Shirley Lamberink and the staff of the Brentwood Animal Clinic (who accommodated Reiki in the care of my pets), Dr. Pam Goble, Dr. Marilyn Komarnisky, Dr. Carol Kujala, Dr. Karen Marsden, Dr. Stephen Marsden, Dr. Heather Steele, and Tina Dienes, animal health technician.

I am indebted to Lorna Savak and Dr. Marnie Wood for longstanding encouragement and support. Thanks also to Heidi Peters, Catherine Potter, and Paul Napora for their guidance.

Peggie Graham and Alison Cheesbrough tirelessly critiqued and edited various drafts of this manuscript. The critical review and comments of Judy Weir, Dr. Pam Goble, Master Inge Saxena, Felicity Edwards, and Pamela Alexander led to great improvements. Many others provided helpful feedback including Lorna Savak's Reiki Circle (Darlene, Dee, Grace, and Valerie), and Natalia's Flower Essence Group (Bev, Jaime, and Joy).

There is one more individual who deserves credit: Natalia's husband, Dr. Bill MacDonald, has provided both of us with moral and financial support that have made writing this book possible.

Susan Mack
on behalf of herself and Natalia Krawetz
Sherwood Park & Edmonton, Alberta, Canada

Part One:

Practising Pet-Oriented Reiki

Chapter 1

Introducing Reiki

Touch is the most basic connection between two living beings. Without it, mammals could not survive. Human babies who are not regularly cuddled and carried, fail to thrive and are unable to connect fully with other human beings. Kittens depend on the touch of their mother's tongue to keep them safe: triggering their ability to eliminate waste and erasing smells that would attract predators. Puppies latch on to their mother's teats for life-nourishing milk, as well as for warmth. Touch keeps us alive, helping each of us to become fully functioning.

Touch is a form of communication. We usually think of it as a physical act, requiring direct contact between those who share it. Its message is carried by the body parts involved, and by the pressure and temperature of the exchange. Compare the differences between the message of care conveyed by gently stroking a cat's fur with that of anger transmitted from a human palm coming down hard across a dog's muzzle. We feel touch on levels beyond the physical exchange: on the emotional level, as we react to the impact of that touch with our feelings, and on the spiritual level as well. When we send prayers for our beloved pet's recovery from illness, we touch spirit solely through conscious intent; and in response, spirit touches our pet and then ourselves. This act of spiritual connection shows that we don't necessarily need physical contact to have an impact on another being.

Touch has therapeutic value; and every mammal instinctively uses it in this way - whether it be through mutual grooming or massage for relaxation, licking to clean a wound or soothe a sore spot, or cuddling up for comfort. All human cultures have some form of touch for therapeutic use. While some have been developed for human beings to care for each other, many can be shared between

humans and other animals, between humans and plants, and sometimes between animals themselves. This book is about one such form of touch, called Reiki.

Reiki is a Japanese term for Universal Life Energy, the vital life force that flows in and around all living things. To transmit Reiki you must be initiated by a Reiki Master. This involves a period of instruction as well as receiving attunements. An attunement is a way in which the Master opens up your inborn, though dormant, ability to draw Reiki energy through your body from outside yourself, and direct it toward a being. That energy then moves to the area that needs healing.

There are two basic forms of Reiki: *hands on* or Level One and *distance* or Level Two. With *hands on*, the palms of the sender are in direct contact with the body of the receiver. With *distance*, Reiki is sent toward the receiver without bodily contact. In any case, there is no manipulation of body tissue; the physical body is touched only gently, if at all.

The purpose of Reiki is to heal. The end result of a good Reiki session is the same for both humans and pets:

- support for the recovery from illness, injury, surgery, and trauma;
- pain management (often to the point that medications can be reduced or discontinued);
- relief from the discomfort of chronic conditions such as arthritis and hip dysplasia;
- comfort during palliative care; and
- help with the transition from this world, for both the dying and their loved ones.

In holistic terms, healing triggers the body's natural impulse toward balance. It is restorative, not necessarily curative. While Reiki does not replace medical care and the practitioner does not diagnose or prescribe, it can complement virtually any form of treatment a being may receive.

Each year thousands of people around the world become Reiki students. Most are interested in it to reduce their own stress, manage their own pain, or help them relax. Most will continue to focus on themselves for the rest of their lives, occasionally sharing Reiki with

family members and close friends. Some will become practitioners providing Reiki as a business. Unless they are allergic to or terrified of animals, most will be asked, at some time, to share Reiki with a pet.

For those who are comfortable sharing Reiki with humans, the experience of working with a pet can be bewildering because what makes sense for sharing with humans doesn't seem to apply. For example, a good Reiki session for a human usually takes place in a comfy chair or on a massage table, in a quiet room with dim lighting and soft music. The person has some idea about the process involved and has consented to participate. Most recipients speak of Reiki in glowing terms: the gentleness of the touch, the sense of safety because they are fully clothed, the deep relaxation while resting comfortably in a soothing environment, the easing of pain. If we can accept that a good Reiki session offers the same benefits whether the recipient is human or animal, why then is a session with a pet different?

There are several reasons. The idea of a massage table or candles holds no sway for pets. In most cases, the pet has no opportunity for consent and is suddenly confronted by a traveling pair of hands invading his personal space. The set hand positions taught for humans don't apply. If you put your hands over the eyes of most animals, they will shrink in fear. Touch a sore spot, even gently, and you may get bitten. Share Reiki with a nervous animal and you may end up with urine on your clothes. And where exactly do you put your hands on a fish? These are a few of the challenges you face when you work with pets.

To where then, do you go for help? Most Reiki Masters, those responsible for initiating others to Reiki, have little experience with pets and pet-oriented Reiki literature is sparse. So not surprisingly, many people find working with a pet to be an unsatisfying experience. As one practitioner said, "I was asked to work with a cat. She looked as if receiving Reiki was something she was enduring.

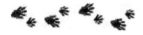

After 10 minutes she left the room and never returned. I'm sure she was uncomfortable and I didn't know what to do about it."

I have found that the best way to learn exactly what pets want and exactly how pets benefit, is from the pets themselves. Building up a solid base of experience means working with many pets of different species, some of whom receive several sessions through time. In time, rules of thumb that can help the healing process become apparent.

Each pet-oriented Reiki session is not only about healing; it is also a spiritual encounter. Being open to these encounters is the first step in transforming a relationship with a pet to one of partnership and intimacy. My journey toward this end has followed a path set by Reiki, as directed by pets. I walk it everyday with commitment and love. It still amazes me that such a simple practice deepens my relationship with animals in ways I didn't think possible, while putting me in touch with larger truths. Please join me on this sacred adventure.

Chapter 2

Developing a Pet-Oriented Partnership:

Lessons in Attention

When people find out that I share Reiki with pets, they are intrigued. If they are familiar with energy work, they may wonder how I get a cat to lie belly-up on a massage table, or ask about the kind of music dogs prefer as background for their sessions. Because most interested pet lovers ask what a pet-oriented Reiki session would look like, I've devoted this chapter to satisfying their curiosity.

A Reiki session is an energetic conversation. The pet initiates the dialog and I respond using my hands and addressing her body. By paying attention to how each of us reacts to what is shared, we become more sensitive to the nuances we communicate. In time, we form a partnership.

Pets have taught me to adjust my response to fit the moment, using a form of improvisation that emphasizes the quality of attention I bring to the process. My biggest lessons in this kind of Reiki conversation are to take my signals from the pet and to treat every situation uniquely. I want to show this at work during a typical session with a dog called Maxine, a German Shepherd.

Maxine had been an animal shelter graduate with a history of physical and emotional abuse resulting in a skittish nature and a tendency to bark. With love and patience her new family helped to heal her, even building a safe room in the basement where she stayed when they left the house so she wouldn't feel overwhelmed and destroy the furniture. She was seven years old when physical problems began to surface for which veterinary care was needed: hip dysplasia and arthritis. I was asked to improve her quality of life with Reiki.

Knowing that Maxine was timid and somewhat skittish, I was a little apprehensive about our first meeting. She set the mood with her first greeting - a loud series of barks warning me to keep my distance. I showed that I'd heeded her warning by starting slowly. We had another contributor at that session: Maxine's person, who sat beside her and calmed her down, thereby ensuring that the tone of our interaction would not escalate beyond Maxine's level of comfort. Everything in this situation suggested a cautious approach, to which I added my voice. Talking slowly and softly, I told her about Reiki: how it was her friend and would let her be in control, and how it couldn't hurt her even if I wanted it to, because Reiki wouldn't allow it. This is my basic introductory talk to any new client, and its delivery in soft, slow tones has a calming effect.

I began to move my hands in rhythm with my voice, giving her gentle strokes. As she relaxed into this, I responded by putting one hand on her body to share Reiki with her. She told me of her pain and her need for vigilance, through her reactions to my moves. Pain was manifested in the sensitive areas along her spine and into her hips. When my hand moved to them she would pull back, so I responded by hovering my hand a few inches above her instead of being in direct contact. At the same time, her person responded with reassurance, scratching her ears to keep her somewhat distracted. Then Maxine relaxed and her eyes started to close. She'd take me by surprise when she'd jerk herself awake so as not to miss anything, showing me the importance she placed on being vigilant. This watchfulness surfaced from time to time because she felt responsible for guarding the house. So I told her that anyone who worked as hard as she did, was allowed to take a break; and we both settled back down. Like all first visits, I had scheduled an hour and a half for the session. Two hours later Maxine let me know that the session had come to a close by drifting off to sleep, and I left.

By the second session, we were creating a dialog in two parts: a greeting ritual followed by our main discussion. First, Maxine would meet me at the door with a welcome bark and then I would give her a treat. I'd try to save it for after the session but she wanted payment up front. Then we'd begin the second part, the main discussion or Reiki session. She would set the pace, letting me place my hands where I felt they belonged most of the time. Sometimes she would guide them, often to places too sensitive for touch and I'd have to move them slightly. As her ailments progressed over the years, she was so sore that I switched entirely to *distance* or non-contact Reiki.

A few sessions into our relationship, Maxine developed a formal conclusion to mark the end of our work for the day. When the session was over, she would throw her favorite toy at me and then

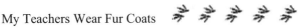

walk me to the door. So, like any visit between friends, our time together had three parts: a greeting ritual, then a deeper exchange, followed by a conclusion. We kept in touch between appointments by *distance*, aided by her photo.

We had a lot of energetic conversations that year, giving me time to observe the changes that resulted. When we first met, Maxine's worried, nervous countenance made her look twelve rather than her actual age of seven years. With Reiki, she became more playful and seemed younger than she had initially appeared, likely because her pain was under better control. She became more confident, more mobile, and even quite mischievous. Her people vacillated between being positively impressed by these changes and wondering what they'd gotten themselves into. As the benefits of Reiki manifested and Maxine began to blossom, our visits became bimonthly unless otherwise needed.

What happened with Reiki was strictly between itself and Maxine. I was only its transmitter. Yet all three of us were joined in this together: Reiki, Maxine, and me. We were partners. As always, Reiki went where it was needed and Maxine chose whether or not she wished to receive it. I could neither force her to accept it nor force it to benefit her; but I could influence her receptivity to it, by paying attention. From Maxine I learned the value of attention, for her watchful presence embodied the alert state. If she could speak English, she would say, " Get up on your haunches, perk up your ears, and watch carefully." She taught me that attention was the key to discovering how to conduct a pet-oriented Reiki session, for she made it clear that my task was to transmit Reiki to her in the way she could best receive it. In exchange, I helped her add a dimension of calm to her vigilance. When we both relaxed and focused on the present moment, we improvised energetically in a way that yielded beautiful results.

If you watched me share Reiki with Maxine, you might wonder what was actually going on. You would see me near the dog, placing my hands on her body or, at times, not being in physical contact with her at all. The session could look like a rip off of the highest order, for there is nothing spectacular in the way it is done and the results may be subtle, occurring even days later. Maxine and I looked like

9

we were just sitting around. In fact, she was working with Reiki in her body. I too, was working - not to bring her Reiki, for it flows of its own accord, but rather to help her receive it. We were both paying careful attention.

In reflecting on my work with Maxine and others, I see that my past experience in the hospitality industry, as a professional chef and restaurant owner, polished my skills in areas directly transferable to pet-oriented Reiki. Reiki is a form of energetic nourishment. Serving it alone would be sufficient to sate the appetite. But think how much more this meal is enhanced if I see myself as the host and invite the pet, as an honored guest, to share that meal. The difference between simply setting food down and sharing a memorable dining experience, is in the details.

Before we actually meet, I prepare by taking account of what I know of his concerns and preferences. And then when we are together, I treat him with an eye to his comfort, extending courtesy and remaining sensitive to his needs. To enhance his enjoyment, I need to be vigilant throughout the meal, taking care of everything in a seemingly effortless way. All of these qualities - consideration, courtesy, sensitivity, and vigilance - are aspects of attentive service, be they as the host at a dinner table or as a Reiki practitioner with a pet. So I will spend the balance of this chapter on these qualities and their contributions to an optimal Reiki session.

Like anyone working with pets, my first contact is usually with that pet's person when he calls for an initial appointment. From his responses to specific questions, I get background information that can set the foundation for my understanding of the pet's preferences and concerns. This data gathering exercise is based on four questions.

- *What kind of pet is involved?*
Obviously it helps to know the species to which the pet belongs. If I will be working with a cat or dog like Maxine, I expect that we will be in physical contact at some point. A fish, however, would be a different matter, and species unfamiliar to me are likely to receive *distance*. Moreover, some breeds of dogs and cats have specific characteristics worth taking into consideration. For example, German

10

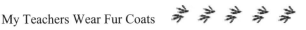

Shepherds, like Maxine, can be protective of their people and homes. By taking this protective nature into account, I prepare myself for the likelihood that she will respond best to a slow and cautious approach. If Maxine had been a Siamese cat, then I would also proceed slowly but for a different reason. These cats tend to be emotionally volatile, suggesting that I should be prepared to be swatted and cursed if the session is not to their liking. We all associate particular species and breeds with particular characteristics: dogs with loyalty and cats with independence, for example. And while I have learned a lot from talking with pet lovers and working directly with pets, reading about animal behavior and the characteristics of breeds has given me information I can use to prepare for our meeting, as well.

- *What is the pet's temperament?*

Most of the animals I work with are mixed breeds; yet there can be huge variations in temperament between individuals of the same breed. Take German Shepherds, for example. I have met aggressive ones and ones so friendly as to allow me into their homes without hesitation. And all things being equal, I'd prefer work with, rather than against, a pet's temperament. This means that when there is a pet like Maxine, who is timid and skittish, I need to heed her warning bark and hold back from touching her, or I might get bitten. However, if Maxine were a timid cat, she might be more likely to hide rather than bite when approached, making the possibility of *hands on* contact remote. Yet if Maxine were a very social rabbit, she might be ready to start a full-contact relationship immediately.

- *How is the pet's health?*

Maxine's health problems, hip dysplasia and arthritis, meant that touch would be excruciatingly painful in certain areas and at certain times. I needed to be assured that she was receiving veterinary care, for sometimes people think I can replace such services, which I cannot. Even so, it helps

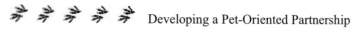

to know if I'll be working with an ill animal who might vomit on my clothes (the reason why I keep a spare change of clothing in my car). If Maxine was recovering from a wound, I'd have to be careful about putting my hands over the affected area. If she had a potentially contagious disease, I'd need to know how long the contagion lasts so I wouldn't spread it to other clients. Regardless, I'd have to wash my hands carefully when her session was over to prevent spreading her germs to other pets.

- *Are there other pets in the household?*

Maxine was the only pet in her household. If she had shared her home with another pet, he, too, might have expected Reiki, even if it was not in the agreement between the pets' person and myself. In this situation, I might add a bit of time for a short session for other, interested pets, to alleviate jealousy or the feeling of being left out.

- *How can I help?*

I knew I was retained to help Maxine manage her pain and since that is within the realm of what Reiki can do, I was happy to be of service. Sometimes the gap between what the pet's person expects and what I can deliver is so large, that the Reiki session is bound to disappoint. In that case, we need to discuss bridging that gap before we begin.

So just like preparing for a dinner party, there are factors I need to take into account - species and breed, temperament, health, and expectations - that have implications for how I will serve a Reiki meal. Taking these into consideration is an exercise in mental preparedness, giving me ideas on how to approach the session.

If I have the time, I'll send some *distance* to the pet in advance of my arrival, so that she will recognize my energetic signature when we meet. Then if we continue our work, as I did with Maxine, I'll ask for a photograph to help me send *distance* at times when I cannot be with her in person.

Advance preparation extends to setting the time and place for our encounter. While the pet's person usually controls the timing of appointments, I suggest that Reiki be shared during the pet's quiet time, rather than when the dog wants to play or the cat is expecting

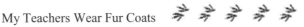

to eat. And although most of my sessions are one hour, I allow 90 minutes for the first meeting so that we have plenty of time for introductions.

When people share Reiki with their pets, I suggest they schedule sessions during the pet's quiet time, as long as the person is calm and relatively stress-free. The worst combination would be trying to share Reiki just after arriving from a rotten day at work and your dog wants to go for a walk. In such a case, neither of you is ready to settle down.

Sometimes the pet's person cannot settle down enough to provide Reiki himself. If you are going through a difficult time or tend to be anxious, high-strung, or emotionally intense, your pet may find Reiki easier to accept when you are doing a self-treatment. Then he can come near you and hitchhike. And sometimes Reiki works best when delivered by a third party.

Pets are more comfortable receiving Reiki in familiar surroundings, which is why I meet them in their homes. If the household situation is a source of their anxiety, Reiki can act as a counter-conditioner, enabling them to relax in circumstances that would usually cause them to tense up. I will, when necessary, visit a veterinary clinic or boarding facility.

Within their home, pets have favorite places where they feel safe and secure. Some are most comfortable on the living room floor in front of the TV watching cartoons. Others prefer to be under a table or on a favorite blanket. And that might mean that I have to stretch my hands across a bed or hunch underneath a table in order to share Reiki with them. But by influencing the timing and location of our meeting, I can extend the courtesy of honoring pet preferences.

And finally, I try to avoid bringing in any trigger that could start our relationship off badly. For example, I keep myself as scent-free as possible, since strong scents are the equivalent of intense light to many species. But careful preparation does not mean that I can slack off when the pet and I actually meet.

Just as the way in which a host receives his guest sets the tone for the occasion, how the pet and I greet each other sets the mood for our work together. Once I'm in his home, I apply what I know about pet etiquette. If he is mobile, we usually introduce ourselves at the front door with a chance to sniff my hand and trouser legs as well as the boots I've discarded at the door, in effect the letters of reference from the previous clients of the day. If he is not mobile, I present my hand for a sniff. Only if it is accepted and he appears calm, do I stroke him. Those animals who recognize my energetic signature from the *distance* I sent in advance of our meeting, often give a bit of a start before settling down.

If the pet appears wary in any way, I proceed more slowly, perhaps starting with *distance*. Then I observe his verbal and nonverbal communication to avoid triggering more fear, nervousness, or aggression. From reading about animal behavior, I learned to look for useful cues:

- Prolonged, direct eye contact is a sign of aggression for many species.

- Dilated pupils that are open more than they should be in the surrounding light conditions, suggest stress or fear, even more so if a cat's ears are flattened and the whiskers are back.

- A cat whose ears resemble steers' horns or whose tail is lashing signals annoyance or worse.

- A cat in the classic Halloween pose with his fur standing on end means, please back off.

- A dog on his back with his tail between his legs lacks confidence.

- A hunched up body might mean pain or excessive fear.

- A growl, especially with a dog's teeth showing, or a cat's hiss, warn me that I am too close and should back off.

Any of these cues tell me that the pet would prefer me to take my time.

I relax into the situation, waiting to make direct, physical contact only after we are acquainted and comfortable with each other. It may take more than one session of *distance* before there is enough trust and comfort for *hands on*, and it is an act of respect to have the patience to wait. While I work with the pet, I tell her about Reiki, what it means to me, and what it might feel like. The soft drone of my voice helps put both of us at ease.

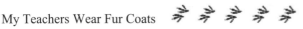

When she is ready for direct contact, I usually start stroking her head with one hand; as she adjusts to this level of contact, I simultaneously float my other hand over her shoulders, then slowly lower it on to her fur. I leave my hands in one place until I sense it is time to move or until she changes position, working slowly towards her rear. This can be a very sensitive area especially for aggressive pets who may store a lot of tension there, so I proceed with caution. It may take several sessions before she will be comfortable enough to allow me to touch this area.

Having her head stroked while receiving Reiki usually distracts a pet, giving her time to adjust to the new sensation of energy work. Seldom do I use two hands (unless the pet is very large) because most seem to be better able to tolerate one-handed Reiki. After that, I let the animal guide my hands to where they are needed, as I will describe later in this chapter.

By this time, I might recognize the rare instance when a pet has rejected Reiki. This was the case with Smoky, a senior cat upset by the presence of Octave, another, newly-adopted senior cat, in his household. The two of them fought at every opportunity and had to be kept in separate parts of the house, a typical result of trying to integrate strange, elderly cats under one roof. I was asked to determine if Reiki sessions would alleviate Smoky's territoriality.

On meeting him, I sensed deep anger and hurt. I began *distance* and immediately sensed an abrupt cut in the energetic flow which I interpreted as his refusal to accept it. Every time I tried to send him Reiki, and I did so on four, separate occasions, I'd be met with the same result. I came to understand that Smoky felt righteous in his anger over the intruder forced on him by the humans in the household, and that he preferred to remain angry about it. I advised his person and the sessions ended until years later, when he became physically ill. This time he was more than ready to accept Reiki and we shared many sessions. Unlike Smoky, most pets I meet are interested in receiving Reiki.

While the pet may welcome my hands, sometimes both hands or even one, is just too much. As Maxine taught me, this sensitivity can vary with the pet or with time, sometimes even within a session. Some pets are fine with direct, *hands on* contact. Others, largely cats,

15

reject immediate *hands on* and prefer that we start with *distance*; only when they are sufficiently relaxed is *hands on* allowed. Even then, many cat clients prefer having their heads stroked with one hand while receiving Reiki through the other; two hands are just too much. There are some pets who prefer *distance*. While both *hands on* and *distance* are equally effective, their acceptance depends on the pet and the situation. Then there are those, in multi-pet households who like to hitchhike, sitting close by when Reiki is being sent to others.

Because Reiki is transmitted by hand, people assume that either there is an approved set of hand positions for pets or I can read a pet's mind about placement. However, I learn placement through vigilance, by constantly monitoring the pet's reaction to where my hands are located on his body. In this way, I noticed that Tabby, a white Cockapoo, would push my hands into position on her chest and throat to receive Reiki. After a while, she would shift her body so that my hands would change position and she'd have me do her back and sides. Wye, a self-possessed, black and white Greyhound, likes receiving Reiki on her bum. So her advice to me is simple: "No matter what the problem, just Reiki my bum, Susan, and everything will get better." And who am I to argue, since she is bigger than me?

Learning hand placement from aquarium fish was very instructive. I usually placed my hands against the tank's glass. Then one day I noticed a sick fish in the tank so I sent *distance* to him. To my surprise, he was attacked by another fish. It dawned on me that by sending Reiki only to him, I was disturbing the balance in the school; it made him different and difference was attacked. So I started to send Reiki to the school as a whole - treating the tank and every being in it, together. The sick fish began to interact with the others, no longer staying in the corner with what I interpreted to be expressions of pain.

Like many other species, the school's sensitivity to energy varied. Usually the fish would crowd around my hands on the glass of the tank, seeking the Reiki. But there were days when they'd keep as far away from my hands as possible because the energy was just too much for them. Then I'd switch to *distance* from a few feet away.

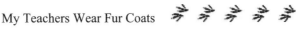

My learning about hand placement has been refined by sharing my home with two cats, Kahlua and Friend, who graciously lend their bodies for Reiki practise when my students visit. Each has a different teaching style.

While Kahlua allows *hands on* contact with her lustrous fur, she is very particular about where those hands are placed. She communicates with her body, frowning at the hand until it is moved to the right place as if to say, "Come on now. Figure it out." If the person doesn't catch on, she will move until the right body part is in contact with the hands and then settle in, moving again as need be. Sometimes she communicates with her voice, squealing or speaking Siamese to say, "Get your hands off that spot real fast!" When she is finished, she delivers a quick swat to say that the session is over.

This is such a contrast to Friend who has the patience of Job. She allows hands to cover every part of her body in succession, before gently yet firmly saying that she is done. To signal that the session is over, she will shift her body away from those hands and look the person directly in the face. Then if those hands are pulled away, Friend settles back down. If they remain in place, she gets up and walks away. So while the hand placements for particular dogs, schools of fish, and specific cats may vary, each individual pet has preferences which can be learned by being vigilant.

Beyond the issue of hand placement, is that of hand pressure. When I started practising Reiki, I was tempted to rest my hands firmly on the pet's body as if this would help push the Reiki through. Yet gentleness is called for, especially on sore, mistrustful, or fragile bodies. If there is a wound or known area of soreness, I'm careful not to touch it directly, unless invited to do so by the pet, though I never touch an unhealed, open wound because of the risk of infection. In such cases, I float my hand above the area or switch to *distance*. I've found that it takes experience and confidence to trust that Reiki will go to where it is needed even if my hand is elsewhere.

Going beyond the intricacies of hand placement is the need to watch over the process as the session unfolds. The pet's schedule for accepting both Reiki and myself is very individual, varying from day to day. As the session proceeds, a particular pet, like Maxine, may begin to relax. Slowly her head might sink into my lap or her eyes start to close. Purrs or soft snores may follow. Another pet may find it hard to settle down, telling me that I need to let him regroup by switching from two hands to one, or to *distance*. I can support this process by staying calm, breathing slowly, and talking quietly to him. Yet just as often, a pet appears to settle in quickly and after 20 minutes or so, walks away. While I never force a pet to stay still, the pet who walks away does not necessarily mean he is finished with the Reiki session. It may just mean he needs a break to assimilate the energy. A trip to the water bowl, perhaps a short munch on kibble, or a brief saunter in the back yard is all that is needed to bring him back for more.

During or after the Reiki meal, the beverage of choice is water, so I ask that pets be given free access to a fresh supply. They seem to know about its importance in flushing the toxins released by Reiki from their system. However, there are times when the pet doesn't drink enough fluids and intake needs to be monitored, particularly if there are long or repeated sessions of Reiki with short intervals in between. In such cases, I show the pet's person how to check hydration levels. And for cats, who usually don't drink enough water, I take advantage of my cooking experience by recommending that people make cat food pudding, adding water to servings of wet food.

The energetic meal we share usually lasts a full hour, though the Reiki itself will continue its work in the pet's body for much longer than that. With pets in great need, sessions can last for several hours, schedule permitting. And when the session is over, some pets and I observe a closing ritual before I leave.

Every energetic meal I serve is different. By paying attention to my pet guests, I have been guided through the subtle variations between individual preferences and across sessions. They have challenged me to extemporize, adapting my approach to them as individuals, to the individual session, and even to shifts moment by moment within that session. They know where they want Reiki and if I pay careful attention, they will tell me where that is - even those for whom direct touch is not possible. They even tell me when they are not interested.

I believe that the attention I pay to this act of hosting adds value to our experience of this energetic meal. I could serve the food and

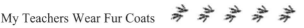

invest nothing else of myself in the experience of sharing it. Many people believe that is enough - to just start the flow and let the rest of the transaction be strictly between Reiki and the pet. As such, it reduces my role to one so passive and detached, that I become just a pair of hands accompanied by the positive, healing intent with which I was originally initiated into Reiki. Or I could choose to prepare carefully for the energetic meal and serve it by rote, making sure everything is in order while letting my mind drift. That, too, would provide Reiki but without any meaningful relationship between the pet and myself. So I have made a third choice, viewing the session as a way in which Reiki, the pet, and I can speak to each other. By adding the qualities of attention to the way I transmit Reiki, I treat my pet clients as cherished guests whom I hope will become true friends. I know they have things to teach me and I am ready to learn in the Reiki session that is our class. A task as important as this one deserves the deepest attention - careful consideration, courtesy, and sensitivity, along with a relaxed state of vigilance.

As I learn to apply these qualities of attention to the preparation for and sharing in our session, I've come to understand that Reiki works in relationship, connecting itself, the pet, and me to each other. Within the context of that session, we teach and learn by responding to what the other presents, just like the host and guest sharing a meal. This simple act of attending to each other in the moment, unfettered by reveries from the past or daydreams of the future, becomes a sacred encounter. It enables us to discover a great deal about each other and provides the place for partnership.

Chapter 3

Engaging in the Reiki Process:

Lessons in Abundance

Transmitting and receiving Reiki looks like a passive process. I merely sit with my hands on the pet's body, or cupped in front of me to transmit across space; in response, the pet does whatever he wishes. Until he shows that he has benefited from our sessions in some way, it is easy for the observer to believe that nothing is happening. I want to dispel this notion by describing some of the different ways in which we are actively engaged.

When I was initiated to Reiki, I became its channel or transmitter. My role is to ensure that Reiki is sent through me to the receiving being, as clearly as possible. All the energetic debris of daily life - emotions like jealousy, anger, impatience, and physical barriers like the flu and my overindulgence in chocolates - can interfere with my ability to transmit Reiki energy. When this happens, the flow from my hands becomes a trickle. The only way to turn the tap back on is through regular self-treatment. While everyone involved in Reiki agrees that self-treatments, that is, giving Reiki to yourself, are the foundation of the practice, not everyone is diligent in maintaining them. In my own experience, self-treatments enable me to ride through the emotional drain of dealing with the myriad issues surrounding the care of pets; keeping things in perspective. So I do myself and my clients no favor by scrimping on this facet of Reiki practice.

When I view my role as strictly one of transmission in the narrowest sense of the term, I see myself as a pair of hands on a body initiated to Reiki. I am merely a conduit; the fundamental relationship is between Reiki and the receiving pet. This visual image reminds me that when I arrive for a Reiki session, I should check my ego at the door. That way, I can let Reiki and the pet decide how they wish to proceed. I have learned, through tragic errors I will describe in other chapters, what happens when I try to

21

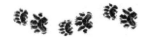

intervene too much - for example, by *repeatedly* directing Reiki *solely* to a particular body site rather than letting that be a matter between the energy and the pet. Yet instead of learning to keep out of the Reiki process as much as possible, I have discovered a fine balance between letting things take their course and actively creating a safe context for the pet. I take my cues from the pet, for he would not want to have anything to do with the Reiki I transmit, if I was not attentive to his concerns and preferences.

In the course of learning the pet's cues, I have also learned how to determine what form of Reiki fits his situation best. While *hands on* is the most well-known form of Reiki, it suits situations where I am able to be with the pet in person *and* he is interested in receiving it *and* he is comfortable enough to allow touch. This leaves a number of situations where *hands on* is not appropriate and thus *distance* is required:

• To introduce myself to a pet before meeting in person; or to keep in touch when I cannot be with him. This is how I keep in touch with my own pets during my working day.

• Emergencies while en route to a pet in need.

• When the pet is in so much pain that *hands on* would overwhelm him.

• Situations, such as open wounds, where direct touch is unsafe because of the chances of infection.

• Introducing highly anxious pets to Reiki so they can relax enough to try *hands on*.

• Emotional conditions like abuse where the pet fears being touched.

• Situations where I am at risk from physical harm. If a dog would rather bite me than experience *hands on*, I use *distance* and watch his response. Sometimes he will then allow me to move to *hands on* before the session is over. But it could take several *distance* sessions first. It's all a judgment call based on what he is willing to tolerate and accept.

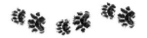

In addition to decisions about whether to use *hands on* or *distance*, I am also faced with decisions related to those pets - often with advanced chronic or terminal illnesses - whose Reiki requirements extend to several hours a day. At first, I would proceed with the session for however long it would take and visit daily, if permitted. Contrary to concerns that such extensive sessions would overload them, I found pets to be fine as long as they were free to walk away from *hands on* or energetically turn off a *distance* session. When they had enough Reiki, they pulled away or started to growl. But if they kept shifting new parts of their bodies to be under my hands, I took this as a signal to continue.

This is quite different from my understanding of what happens when people receive extended Reiki sessions. Some may suffer an overload because they are ungrounded, disconnecting the energetic exchange from their bodies to the world outside. In such cases, energy becomes trapped inside them and they may report feeling spacey, suddenly having a headache, or feeling like they are going to burst, perhaps in anger. In my experience, most pets are able to release any excess energy out their paws and into the room. One exception was Katie, a cat who I felt to be floating above her body. By having her person Reiki her paws, she was then able to become and remain grounded.

As my practice continued, the needs of pets with extensive, daily Reiki requirements overwhelmed my schedule. Then I learned about the healing attunement, a shorter, more intense form of Reiki developed in North America. This works for *some* terminally ill pets whose Reiki requirements have escalated to three or more hours of Reiki a day, or for *some* chronically ill pets who have similar needs. But frail or old pets can become frightened or upset by healing attunements; they hide, have dilated pupils, or act skittish. While I continue to use the healing attunement when necessary and appropriate, I do so with great caution. It is very important to carefully monitor a pet's reaction to such intervention, for it cannot be used in all cases.

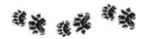

As I continued to share Reiki with pets, I learned more about the nature of their participation. When I first started, I thought of the pet as the passive partner, allowing Reiki to do whatever it chose. I didn't know what went on in the pet's body as he worked with the Reiki; that was strictly a matter between them. I soon became aware of how much the pet influenced his receipt of Reiki through expressing his concerns and preferences. And for a long while, I thought I understood the pet's role completely. While I tried in many ways to respect the pet's wishes, I believed he was limited to expressing them within the confines of the session. As with myself, I saw the pet as actively engaged in the Reiki process, within defined limits. Once the session was over, he might continue to work with any Reiki he had received; but the interaction between the Reiki triad (Reiki, myself, and the pet) was over.

Pets taught me that they can actively engage Reiki in many different ways. One of my most memorable lessons in pet participation was on the concept of energetic directing - that a pet could direct exactly where he would receive Reiki. When my Siamese cat, Beakers, needed help I asked several friends to send him Reiki. One would send *distance* but another reported his preference for a form of energy therapy called Therapeutic Touch. The friend who sent him Reiki told me that Beakers had her concentrate on his face. If she attempted to direct her hands to any other part of his body, he refused to accept Reiki. So the face it was. In talking with the friend who sent him Therapeutic Touch, she told me that Beakers enjoyed it over his body from the neck down. When she attempted to go to his face, he refused it. The mystery was solved when I realized that both women were sending to him at the same time. Clearly he decided to have the best of both worlds. I always knew that pets who accepted Reiki worked with it in their body; but until this happened with Beakers, I did not appreciate the extent to which they could direct its path. While I have never experienced this phenomenon again, I know that it is possible.

The more common phenomena I've learned from pets are the ways in which they can engage Reiki through me, beyond our appointed time together: energetic calling and energetic blocking. As

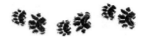

I developed a regular clientele, pets would call me energetically to request Reiki if they needed it, when I was sending *distance* to someone else. If we had worked together intensively or for a long time, they memorized my energetic phone number and felt free to use it. They'd interrupt the energetic line connecting me to the receiver of a particular *distance* I was sending, just like the call waiting feature on a telephone. So I refer to this as energetic calling.

My first such experience was with Higgins, a strikingly handsome orange cat who suffered from painful bouts of pancreatitis (inflammation of the pancreas). I would be sending *distance* to someone else and his image would come to mind. I'd ask him to wait, his image would recede, and I'd make sure to fit him in next. If he believed he was waiting too long, his image would re-surface as a reminder that he'd appreciate Reiki as soon as possible.

Since then, I've learned that pets can dial my energetic number in different ways. While some send me an image, others, like Ginger, send a breeze in the middle of my forehead or specific, relevant bodily sensations. As Ginger's oral cancer progressed, making his mouth profoundly uncomfortable, I would know he was calling me when my own mouth would start to feel swollen and my tongue and lips would go numb. I would then call his person, who had a range of prescribed homeopathic medicines to be used under specific circumstances. She would dose him with whatever medication most fit the bodily sensations I would be experiencing, and he would then relax.

Ginger also participated in teaching me that I could sometimes receive energetic calls from more than one pet at a time. Once, he and Smoky, another cat client, contacted me at the same time. I knew who was on my line because my face felt as if it had split in two: each half had different, specific sensations - the left side mimicked Ginger's symptoms while the right, Smoky's; and each cat needed Reiki now. I was pleased that they felt free to call me no matter what the need, because it meant I was their trusted friend.

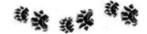

As I became more experienced at responding to energetic calls, my sensitivity became so refined that I can now receive them at any time, whether or not I'm sending Reiki. Once, I was driving from an appointment when I felt a sense of urgency and pain coming from a source that I could not identify. So I listened to the messages on my answering machine for clues. There was a message: "We're going to the hospital" - no name, phone number, or any identifier. I called several people whose pets it might have been and none fit the bill. Finally, I just sent *distance* with the intention that it go to the being who needed it. Immediately I got a sensation of excruciating mouth pain and knew who it was - a feline client 200 miles away who was recovering from dental surgery. Apparently her pain killer had worn off and her people were without additional medication. I responded with Reiki and she started to settle down en route to the veterinary clinic for help. By the time they arrived at their destination, she was no longer in distress.

Energetic calling is now part of my understanding of a pet's Reiki repertoire. I believe it is an example of parity between the pet and myself. The pet has a need and I help fill it. And because we are friends, we have a mutual understanding that I will be there for him when he needs me, even if it is after hours. As our intimacy deepens, he becomes more willing to call me at his most vulnerable times. When his need becomes urgent, he may use energetic blocking - deliberately diverting to himself all *distance* I may be sending at the time.

My first teacher of energetic blocking was my cat, Christmas Blessing. Blessing suffers from chronic ailments with which he lives in constant pain. When the weather changes, his pain can escalate to the point where he takes action. I might be doing a self-treatment and he will come in the room. Suddenly, I'll feel the flow to myself turn off completely and go to him. This was well beyond the energetic calling that I knew. He taught me that an animal in dire need calls me in a different way, as if he knows I have two special numbers: one for most energetic calls and another for Reiki 911. When he dials 911 energetically, he diverts all Reiki to himself and blocks any

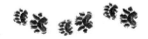

distance being sent to others, just like my feline friend Ginger did after dental surgery.

Ginger's recovery was very painful because his kidney disease prevented the use of painkillers. So for the next three days, he took remedial action by transferring any *distance* Reiki I attempted to send to any other being, as if he had energetic call forward. And he taught his companions - several dogs and one cat - how to do this as well.

I have also learned that need, not size, is the source of the pet's ability to block. For example, Gottfreid, a 12-pound Bichon, was perfectly capable of diverting Reiki that was being sent to Maxine (the German Shepherd in Chapter Two) when his need for it exceeded hers.

Blocking flew in the face of what I knew about Reiki and pets. It seemed as if a pet in deep distress could enter my energetic field and take Reiki for himself without so much as "I beg your pardon." I thought that blocking was an abuse of our friendship, as I felt invaded by a force I couldn't control. I started to retaliate with interventions of my own.

When blocking would happen, I would disconnect the *distance* I was sending and try again. But it didn't make any difference. Then I would focus my will as strongly as possible to send that *distance* to the pet for whom it was intended. That didn't make any difference either. In time, I learned that the only effective action I can take is to disconnect from the *distance* I am sending as soon as possible, so I can connect with the blocker, and arrange for others to send *distance* to blockers when I need to send *distance* to someone else. It took me some time to appreciate blocking, for I felt powerless against a rather rude and pushy pet, even if he did need Reiki.

Now I understand the phenomenon more fully. The pet who calls me on the 911 energetic line needs help fast. And so my wishes, valid though they may be, are overridden much the same as if I was pushed out of my car as it was commandeered for a police chase. The pet's circumstance is so dire that he needs all the Reiki he can

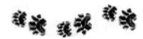

get; and so Reiki provides it, by allowing whatever Reiki I transmit to be all of the Reiki I *can* transmit at that time. In retrospect, it is obvious that the cord connecting the pet with Reiki is strong and direct. Once established, it remains in place so that it can be used as required.

These phenomena - energetic directing, energetic calling, and energetic blocking - have shown me that pets play a far more active role in the Reiki process than I would have thought possible. They can control the Reiki they receive; they can request it without depending on their person to arrange a session; and they can divert it when they are in dire need. To me these actions are proof of the pet's engagement in the Reiki process.

I also noticed that these three phenomena only occur during *distance* sessions. They have never happened with *hands on*. As a result, I believe that the nature of the connections between *hands on* and *distance* are different. The energetic linkage in *distance* enables it to be interrupted or diverted by a determined receiver - even though that receiver may not be the one for whom the Reiki was originally intended.

I accept the existence of lasting linkages between Reiki, the pet, and myself and the idea that they can be engaged at any time, without my initiation. Then I was introduced to two other phenomena that extended my knowledge about the nature of energetic linkages even further. My teachers were pets in multi-pet households.

I mentioned in the previous chapter the need to make short sessions available to other household pets, when I'm there for their companion. This mitigates any curiosity or concerns about jealousy or dominance in the household hierarchy. Since I was taught only to direct Reiki to one being at a time, doing some short sessions on the side worked well. Then one day when I was sharing Reiki with my sister, the family dog, Scruffy, wanted some at the same time. He wasn't prepared to wait and the look he gave me was more than I could bear. So I put a hand on each of them and felt the flow divide. In my mind's eye, I saw a gold band of Reiki dividing itself in size and intensity so that it could be shared. Scruffy got the most, so I

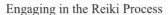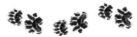

assumed he was in the most need of it, and my sister got what was left. Reiki showed me that in the context of a session there is some for every one present, according to need. Now, when other pets in the household can't bear to wait their turn, I share Reiki with those in the room who want it, by putting one hand on one pet and one on the another, or even by using the soles of my feet (since these are the four contact points from which Reiki can be accessed).

Household companions instinctively know there is enough Reiki to go around, even if they feel no need to come directly to me asking for a portion. They know that as Reiki fulfills the pet's needs, it is abundant enough to extend itself to include whoever else is sharing the space. I've noticed this most during lengthy or intensive sessions, where Reiki coming from the palms of my hands or soles of my feet and/or the paws of the pet receiving it, starts to fill up the room and benefit others. Often, humans who are in that room report a feeling of relaxation as the session proceeds, and other pets who take advantage of the overflow quiet down and show signs of relaxation: lying down, resting, or sleeping. When the healing energy permeates the room, the atmosphere becomes calm and peaceful. I call this phenomenon of tapping into the Reiki overflow, hitchhiking, and it can happen whether I am sharing *hands on* or *distance*. Whatever Reiki is not needed by the receiving being permeates the rooms in which I, as transmitter, and the pet, as receiver, are located; and those beings in the vicinity of either of us can hitchhike on it. My pets enjoy the *distances* I send to other pets from home, because they can hitchhike on the excess that flows from my access points (my palms and soles). I have no doubt that those in the vicinity of the receiving pet also get the benefit of his Reiki (flowing out from his paws).

I still remember visiting Sophie, a tortie cat made anxious by the lengthy absence of her people. She needed Reiki but wanted nothing to do with my hands, so I went to the far edge of the room and sent her *distance*. Peanut, her feline companion, and then Hazel, the family rabbit, lined themselves up along the energetic axis between

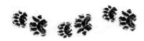

Sophie and myself, to enjoy the session as well; and soon all three began to nod off. From this kind of experience, I get a message from Reiki saying that there is more than enough for all who need it, and that the act of healing the pet heals his living space as well. Reiki has an abundance of energetic fibers that it generously extends throughout the session space, so that everyone there benefits. In multi-pet households, Reiki taught me that its energetic cords build a healing network that extend through palms, soles and paws, beyond the pet and myself.

Working with pet-oriented Reiki has expanded my understanding of its fundamental right to work with the pet on its own terms. Yet I've learned that my role is an active one in this process: ensuring that I clearly transmit Reiki, and deciding on the manner of that transmission as I respond to the pet's concerns and preferences. At times, I overstep these boundaries and wish to do more - for I still have to refine the art of detaching from the outcome of some sessions. While I know that Reiki will do whatever it is supposed to, there are times when the way it manifests is not the way I would have liked.

I have come to appreciate the many ways in which pets actively participate in Reiki. I now understand that they can initiate a session of their own accord, and that once engaged, they have more control over it than I could have possibly imagined. Beaker's ability to direct energy continues to amaze me. Others introduced me to my distinct energetic signature which they can identify and use to contact me beyond the confines of our sessions together. Pets like Blessing, Ginger, and Gottfreid showed that they can initiate Reiki sessions through energetic calling or blocking. Scruffy taught me how to share. Thanks to pets like Sophie, Peanut, and Hazel, I've seen how Reiki can extend its reach, touching and being touched by all living beings in the vicinity, during a session. These are all teachings that I treasure.

Behind these teachings is an even more important one that has deepened my appreciation of Reiki. It has to do with my implicit assumptions about anything of great value: that something of great worth is rare, difficult to find, and the object of competition. Yet

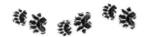

Reiki is far from rare; by its very nature, it exists in and around all living things. It is not hard to find; from experience, I know that it is easily accessed; my only difficulty lies in fully committing to its practice. Being raised in the North American culture of competition - of never having enough and thus always wanting more - I have had to learn that Reiki is not a prize to be won at some other being's expense. Through energetic sharing and hitchhiking, pets have gently guided me away from that competitive misconception by teaching me about Reiki's abundance. Time and again they have simply showed me that when it comes to Reiki, there is always enough to go around.

Chapter 4

Supporting the Healing Journey:

Lessons in Uniqueness

In this chapter I look beyond the fundamental triad in my practice - Reiki, the pet, and myself - to the most significant human who can assist his healing journey: the pet's primary caregiver. Sometimes when a pet and I form a strong healing partnership, his person believes that she is a third wheel. At the darkest times, she may see herself as nothing more than a loving, human wallet - concerned enough for his welfare to arrange for special services, yet lacking a role beyond paying for them. So this chapter is devoted to addressing the question: Where do I, as my pet's caregiver, fit into his healing journey? In response, I will showcase an extraordinary caregiver I named Sylvia, whose exceptional qualities show how a pet's person can contribute significantly to his healing journey. And then I will turn the question back to you, for each caregiver's situation is unique.

Sylvia was the primary caregiver of a delightful, elderly Bichon I have named Gottfreid. Because he enjoyed attention, she would dress him in little outfits and carry him on the main street of town, where they would be stopped by people eager to admire him. She continued this practice as he aged, even when he developed kidney disease and arthritis. For a while, they were able to manage these ailments on their own. Sylvia prepared his favorite Beef Wellington to perk up his appetite, and plugged in the heated pet bed when he seemed a bit stiff. But in time, they needed other help: herbal formulations to ease the load on his kidneys, regular blood work and urinalysis as a basis on which to change his treatment protocol, and Reiki to help manage his pain on a daily basis. So she assembled a team devoted to his care: a conventional veterinarian, a holistic veterinarian, and myself.

Of course, Gottfreid made it clear that he was in charge. He had a strong will to live that enabled him to ride through difficult periods with relative ease and he had a strong interest in his care. If you

watched carefully, he would provide clues not only about how he was feeling, but also about what he wanted. He was also in control of his Reiki. He chose whether or not to accept it. And when he received it, he chose how actively he would work with it in his body.

Gottfreid took advantage of his ability to tap into my energetic signature when it suited him, especially when it involved his favorite Beef Wellington treats. As his illness progressed, his veterinarian advised Sylvia to stop the treats because it was too difficult for his digestive system to handle. Sylvia did, but she forgot to tell me. It also became clear that Gottfried had not been consulted.

About two weeks after his dietary regime had changed, I was driving from his appointment and had a craving for Beef Wellington. "This is strange," I thought. "I don't even like Beef Wellington that much." But I followed my body, stopped at the grocery store, and prepared that dish when I got home. Usually, if this is my own body's craving, one generous helping of that food is enough. But this craving continued.

After two weeks of yearning for and eating Beef Wellington, it occurred to me that this might have something to do with Gottfreid. I asked Sylvia, "When did he last eat Beef Wellington?" Then she told me about the dietary change and I told her how I felt compelled to eat Beef Wellington even though I'm not particularly fond of it. "Might Gottfreid be communicating his wish to eat it too?"

That evening she gave him Beef Wellington and my craving disappeared. And it never came back, because she decided to give him his treat once a week. Sylvia altered the recipe after discussing it with his veterinarian, adamant that Gottfreid be indulged in his advancing years. And since the veterinarian believed that the dog would leave his physical form within six months, he accepted her decision.

While Gottfreid behaved as if his world revolved around him, it did so because Sylvia was devoted to making that happen. She had a keen sense of what was in his best interest. Sometimes that meant he was indulged - with Beef Wellington, for example; other times it meant following veterinary orders to the letter. Sylvia's only concern was ensuring that her dog had the best possible quality of life.

By now it should be obvious that Sylvia and Gottfreid were bound together by a strong cord of love. Gottfreid adored Sylvia and

the feeling was mutual. This bond supported her commitment to him when times got tough. Without it, it would have been all too easy for Sylvia to give up and seek the most expedient and economic solution: euthanasia - well before Gottfreid was prepared to die.

I've learned that their bond was unique, for people are bonded to their pets in varying strengths. I've seen situations of benign neglect, where the pet and his person don't seem to have much to do with one another, other than sharing space. When such a pet is needy, he is often ignored because his person isn't aware of his needs until he becomes very ill. I've noticed differences in the caregiver-pet bond, even within the same household. Bowser may be a family member whose every whim is indulged, but Fluffy may be regarded solely as a mouser whose needs are minimal. Yet having witnessed bonds whose lack of strength is a detriment to the pet's well-being, I also recognize that some strong bonds can be harmful. For example, I have worked with pets whose people are so strongly attached to them that they become emotionally distraught or physically ill when those pets improve, because the balance in the relationship has changed and they are more comfortable with the way things were. And I have witnessed acts of revenge by people who are strongly bonded to aloof pets. If such a pet takes a shine to me, his person might feel rejected, setting the stage for jealousy and often subconscious retaliation, such as forgetting to feed him or reducing essential medications. In such circumstances, caregiver termination of the pet's Reiki sessions is part of the package.

While Sylvia and Gottfreid were strongly bonded and he was a much-cosseted pet, she always kept his best interests at heart. And part of acting in his best interests was to arrange for additional care when his needs became too much for her. For example, when she was queasy about having to give him injections, she hired a veterinary nurse to make house calls instead. It was fortunate that she had the financial means to do so.

While I believe that where you spend your money shows what you care about, priorities can change. The sudden loss of a job or expensive repairs to the family's only vehicle can create hardship as well as the need for a payment plan. Sometimes, if the pet is responding well to Reiki and finances are the only thing getting in the way, I will waive my fees until they are able to be paid, which may mean several years after the sessions are over. Then there are people who are more than financially able but have different priorities when it comes to pet care. I listen as they proudly show me their plasma screen and DVD player or excitedly discuss their Caribbean cruise, yet want my services discounted or discontinued because they choose not to afford them. Fortunately, Gottfreid's care was high on Sylvia's list of priorities. And this was how I learned that level of wealth was not a good predictor of the willingness to continue with services like Reiki; instead, it was the depth of the pet-person bond. Even though she was far from my wealthiest client, she was able to allocate the necessary financial resources.

But loving your dog and being able to pay to get help for him are not the only things needed in the caregiver's repertoire. There are a host of skills and personal qualities that come in handy. Take observational skills, for example. I've known people who haven't noticed that their dog is losing weight or that their cat hasn't eaten in days. Whatever the reason, they often don't respond to these rather obvious signals of distress until the pet is in crisis. Compare this to Sylvia. Having read books and magazines about dogs, she knew what to watch for in Gottfreid's behavior that would mark the signs of an illness or even a veterinary emergency. At times, she would sense when he just wasn't himself, take him to his veterinarian only to be told that he seemed fine, and then two weeks later re-visit that clinic with an obviously sick dog. Over time, his veterinarians grew to respect her ability to sense problems in advance.

Sylvia also knew how to manage and coordinate those she hired as her dog's health care team. She kept all of us informed both of Gottfreid's progress and the results of his visits to the other healing professionals. Thanks to her initiative, those involved in her dog's care communicated with each other. At best, our actions worked together. At worst, they were at cross purposes and we needed to straighten them out, like those Beef Wellington treats, for example. We were able to pull together as a team because Sylvia made it easy for us to do so.

In situations such as this, it isn't unusual for one team member to develop respect for and interest in the findings of another. So I wasn't surprised when one of his veterinarians became interested in the signals I picked up during my sessions and used that information

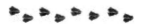

to modify treatment protocols when warranted. This has happened with other clients as well. For example, one day I felt pain in my ear that I knew belonged to Beauty, a cat client. Her veterinarian was interested in the quality of the sensations I had regarding her condition. As a result, he decided against the usual treatment (which may have punctured her ear drum) and dealt with it in another way. So sometimes through Reiki, I become a valued team member working with others for the pet's health, as I did with Gottfreid.

Gottfreid was in an exceptional situation because his person respected Reiki and made an effort to ensure that I was included in professional discussions with the others who provided his care. All to often, I am a neglected adjunct because many veterinarians ignore the presence of Reiki and some pet people don't even mention it, especially if they fear veterinary censure. Some veterinarians believe that Reiki doesn't work, or if it does, its role is not significant. In their opinion, as long as the person has the money, she can proceed with whatever Reiki she wants because it won't make much difference.

After all the work Sylvia had done to make sure that we worked as a team, I was shocked when her new holistic veterinarian suggested that Reiki be stopped once new medical interventions were in place for Gottfreid. He reasoned that since the acupuncture he would use was energetically based, there was no need for another, energetic therapy. I wondered how he would have reacted if our roles had been reversed - with my suggesting that his interventions be discounted because Reiki was in use. Still, Sylvia viewed him as an essential player and started to think he might have a point. So to compromise, I suggested that we cut Gottfreid's Reiki back very slowly and systematically, so we could observe the effect the decrease would have. As we noticed the negative changes that ensued (more restlessness and irritability on his part), we were able to increase the amount of Reiki he received well before he went into crisis. I've found that with chronically ill pets, discontinuing Reiki is a foolish notion. I don't pretend to know exactly what Reiki contributes that other interventions don't or can't, but I do know that substantially decreasing or discontinuing Reiki with such pets may result in a health crisis for them.

Regardless of the amount of Reiki and other medical care he received, Gottfreid started to deteriorate as the years went by. And over time, Sylvia had to stand up to family members and friends who believed she was spending too much money on him. "After all, he is old and has to die sometime," they would say. And if this didn't affect her actions, they would tell her that the treatments he was being given were ineffective, particularly Reiki which they believed to be a sham.

She stopped these conversations by taking a stand - becoming a Reiki student, so she could care of Gottfreid's daily energetic needs. Because of this, we could reduce the frequency of my visits, saving her money in the long run. While I try to encourage people to consider learning Reiki, many are not able to give their pet the regular, consistent sessions Sylvia did; and some become so distraught over their pet's well-being that he is better served by a third party.

Sylvia's deep bond with Gottfreid was expressed by more than money. It was expressed by more than love. She had the skills and temperament to coordinate and manage information, allocate financial resources and deal assertively, yet respectfully, with professionals. Sylvia was command central. But while she sounds like a saint, she was also deeply human.

As Gottfreid aged and his diseases progressed, she became discouraged, for she hoped that medical care and Reiki might have kept him well for much longer. There were times when she was so tired from juggling the many responsibilities of her life apart from Gottfreid, with her desire to be there for him, that she became cranky. Increasingly, she had to weigh the costs of yet another round of blood work against the costs of repairing a leaky porch. She suffered from the feeling that no matter what she did, it was never enough, for she desperately wanted to do everything perfectly - as if by doing so, she could keep his diseases at bay and he would live forever.

I often think about Sylvia when people ask me about the caregiver's role. But I seldom hold her up as an example. Don't get me wrong, I admire and respect Sylvia and everything she did. But having worked with so many pets and their people, I have learned that different caregivers are noteworthy in different ways. And just

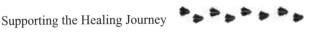

because I think a particular one is exceptional, doesn't mean that everyone should try to emulate her.

At the risk of sounding trite, what I have learned is that every caregiver and every pet-person relationship is unique; no one is perfect. Some, like Sylvia, are bonded to their pets by a strong, abiding love. Others are bonded by a sense of obligation. Some are tied together with chords of co-dependency that threaten to choke them both, while others are hardly bonded at all. I have watched people juggle complex priorities in order to be there for their pets; and I have watched people with relatively simple lives be unable to help their pets in their time of greatest need. Some pets have people who are skilled at care and have the moxie to garner appropriate support. Others find being in a room with a sick pet too distressing to bear on a daily basis; and some of them are unable to think of other solutions for his care. So they live in anguish, either letting the pet linger because they cannot bear to act, or choosing euthanasia to put an end to their own, rather than their pet's, suffering.

As I read this list, it is all too easy for me to judge them. I have my own standards and I sometimes don't meet them. I never knew what qualities, skills, and resources I had, until I called on them. In caring for my own pets, I found myself capable of doing some things I could never have imagined, and disappointed that I couldn't do others I took for granted would be easy to fulfill. At times I have been bewildered, at times cranky, and often tired; all are part and parcel of my commitment to caregiving. I know that it is possible to love a pet deeply and still fall short of providing ideal care, for I have done it.

When people ask me for guidance, instead of holding up an ideal model, I suggest that they ask themselves the following questions:

- What is the strength and quality of my bond to my pet?
- How do I evaluate and juggle my pet's care in terms of competing priorities (financial, temporal, and otherwise)?
- How will my own skills and personal qualities help me to gather resources and support?

- How well do I distinguish between my own needs and those of my pet?

In watching the pet-person relationship unfold at times of great stress, people may take actions of which I don't personally approve or behave in ways that are difficult for me to witness. I am always torn between the self-satisfaction of judging them and the more challenging task of accepting each relationship as it is. I continue to find myself in situations where I'm sure that I know how the pet's person should behave - even when I have no such right. Slowly, I am learning that I can suggest, I can guide, but I cannot control. Sometimes my advice will be heeded; at other times, ignored. But this is how it is and how it will continue to be. Each person's relationship with his pet is unique. They need to work it out, together. And I need to accept it as the context within which I will work and get on with the task at hand - sharing Reiki with his pet.

Part Two:

Improving A Pet's Quality of Life

Chapter 5

Getting Pain Out of the Way: Lessons in Service

Pain is one of the most brutal teachers any being can have. Its descriptors speak volumes about its methods of instruction: the cold or heat of its temperature, the pulsing or aching of its frequency, and its range in intensity - from barely there to unbearable. Those in pain remark on its constant presence, for it is a loyal and exacting teacher. Pain orders a pet to pay attention.

Pets in pain may hunch, whine, yelp, bite, or withdraw. At times, their cues are so unlike ours that we don't recognize them as signals for help. Some bear their pain so stoically that it remains unobserved, even by those closest to them. Regardless of how they react to it, rest assured that pain is front and center. Just as pain preoccupies the affected pet, it overtakes the ability of many caregivers to provide assistance, making them feel helpless. They turn to others, to provide the medication or therapies like Reiki that will make the pain go away. And so, I set about working with pets in pain, trusting that Reiki will be in the pet's best interest.

Sometimes Reiki is all that is needed. Take Cheekie, for example, a ten year old West Highland Terrier who was waiting for medical tests. His veterinarian asked that he be taken off all medications for three weeks, before final testing to confirm a probable diagnosis of lupus. Because Cheekie could hardly move, we shared Reiki to provide him with non-medicated pain management. After five *hands on* sessions in about a week, he was running again and could even jump up on the bed. So his person learned Reiki to keep him comfortable. The diagnosis was not confirmed and we may never know the cause of his distress, but because of Reiki he plays as if nothing has ever been wrong. What Cheekie knows is that Reiki can comfort pets in distress.

Through working with Cheekie and others, I have learned what my role is in pain management. It is not pain killer, because that

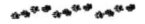

belongs to Reiki. Instead, I am called to be of service - to provide the use of my hands as a transmitter of Reiki energy and by doing so with care, creating a situation within which both the pet and the pet's person can let go of the pain and move on. And so, I will use my own pets as examples as I explore the role of service in pain management, beginning with my dog.

Crackle, known officially as American and Canadian Champion Braewood Tarnished Brass, is an American Cocker Spaniel. She wears a long, black, show coat with a white muzzle and a soft expression on her face. She was pregnant with her last litter when she joined my three-cat household. On her arrival as the latest family member, my cats ignored her and she was able to settle in quietly.

She was restless on her first night, likely because she was in the final stages of pregnancy, at the ripe old age of seven. I couldn't settle down either, worried about my lack of experience with labor and delivery. Finally, we both drifted off to sleep.

I awoke a couple of hours later, aware of a strong, painful pressure toward my right side. Crackle was also up, anxiously staring at me; she, too, was in pain. I immediately understood that the pain I was experiencing was her way of letting me know she needed Reiki, and I began *distance* at once. Soon, the pressure inside me shifted and eased; the puppies had moved into a more comfortable position and settled down, and as this happened, Crackle went back to sleep.

When I indulge in analysis, I can offer the following explanation for what happened. Reiki lowered the anxiety that accompanied the puppies' and Crackle's discomfort, enabling them to shift their focus away from the pain, and thereby restoring their sense of control over their own situation. By relaxing into that situation, they were able to get the pain out of the way and return to the task of slumber. Regardless of the explanation, Crackle began a nightly pattern of wake up calls. In the last two weeks of her pregnancy, these calls happened in the daytime as well.

Crackle delivered five huge puppies: four boys and a girl. I was grateful that mother and children were strong and healthy, but one look at their large sizes told me why she had been so uncomfortable.

In reflecting on our experience, I examined my role in providing them comfort. I was reminded of the Greek word, doula, meaning in

44

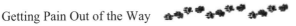
service. A doula is a female whose sole role is to support the mother-to-be before, during, and after birth. She provides comfort and offers ways to relax, giving the expectant mother the chance for a confident and positive birthing experience. Like any close relationship, it hinges on trust and open communication. I came to the conclusion that I was Crackle's doula and, in the process, also served the same role with those puppies - offering Reiki support and pain relief on request. We had a clear communication system: rising pain in my body to signal her need and in turn, her more relaxed behavior as the Reiki began its work. And while our relationship continues, we have both been pleased with her spay surgery. That way, we can both be sure to sleep well through every night.

My cat, Christmas Blessing, is not as fortunate as Crackle. His health challenges are so extensive that all sorts of measures need to work together: mindful care at home, conventional veterinary care, alternative veterinary care, and Reiki. Supported with patience and love, they make the difference between mere existence and his ability to enjoy life.

Our relationship started while I was working with Sara, an elderly cat who received Reiki from me five days a week. He was outside, a known stray whom Sara's people were feeding. One day I looked out the window and saw him standing on the sidewalk gazing at me, and I was washed with a thought that, as in the story of Christmas, here was a stranger in an inhospitable world asking for help. Unlike Mary and Joseph, he would need more than a room for the night. He was caught, kenneled, and taken for immediate veterinary attention for an infection from his war wounds: the scratches and bites of several fights with other tomcats. He was exhausted, sick, and very scared. The veterinarian suggested that with his relatively small size and deteriorating health, he wouldn't have lasted much longer outdoors. After all, he was about three years old, the age at which most long-term strays die.

After being neutered, he came home with me, on Christmas Eve. My female cats, Kahlua and Friend, had to adjust to the presence of male energy. At the time, I thought the adjustment would be temporary, fully expecting to find another home for him. But I quickly learned of the deep emotional scars he bore. Any fast moves on my part terrified him. Anything I picked up was perceived as a

45

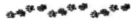

weapon and he would cower, whimper, and shake. He was scared of men and motorcycles. Loud noises gave him the willies. He needed time, patience, and love to help him overcome his fears. Under the circumstances, he could not be put up for adoption. He was mine and I was his, forever.

To become a full-fledged family member, he needed a name. Names have power and I believed that the right name would help him heal. Over the next few days, I tried out many names with no response on his part. Then, one day I was sitting quietly with him, sharing Reiki. Realizing I was hopelessly in love with him, I asked, "Are you my Christmas Blessing?" He purred, my heart melted, and his name was set.

While he enjoyed his new name, he had problems accepting it. Emotionally, he was a basket case of fear, depression, and despair. So, I consulted an animal communicator who said that Blessing had been kicked out of so many homes for spraying that he was mistrustful. While mine was a nice, warm home, he kept waiting for the other shoe to drop: to be thrown out as he had in the past. He felt he wasn't worthy; he was garbage. He was sick enough that death looked welcome and it took solid determination on my part to persuade him otherwise.

Over the next year, Blessing had five hours of *hands on* and *distance* a day, spread over several sessions. His reaction to *hands on* was similar to mine when I was introduced to Reiki: he would freeze into position because of his fear of human contact. Only my faith that Reiki would help him heal kept me continuing with a process that was so scary for him. After several months, he began to enjoy his sessions.

Five months after he had become a family member, I woke up to a veterinary emergency. Blessing was lying under the desk, unwilling to move. He had an acid-alkaline imbalance that produced enough crystals in his urine to block his urethra. Because he couldn't urinate, bodily wastes were re-circulating in his body and poisoning him. Yet again, he was ready to die. Instead, a catheter was inserted into his penis to make it possible for him to urinate and his diet was changed to help dissolve the crystals. A week later, catheter removed, he left the veterinary hospital and came home.

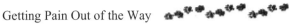

You might wonder why he became so sick when he was receiving so much Reiki. Why didn't it act as a preventative? His veterinarian has a theory about that. In her experience, long-term stray cats often do quite well outdoors until illness or accident kills them, because it is a matter of survival. When they find a good home, the necessity to be so vigilant wears off. And that is such a big change for them, it becomes a source of stress. In other words, Blessing had too much of a good thing and his body just couldn't handle it.

Even change that is welcome (like his being rescued or one of us winning the lottery) is associated with stress. In humans, major stress-related illnesses often strike within two to three years of a highly stressful period. Since cat's lives are comparatively shorter, becoming severely ill five months after being rescued was within the right time frame for Blessing.

Blessing's urinary condition is chronic: it rears its ugly head from time to time. Though dietary changes have helped to keep it at bay, any stressor can set it off. To compound the situation, he gets bacterial infections, possibly associated with osteomylitis. An unusual pelvic formation also contributes to the problem. No wonder that more than Reiki is needed to get him back on track.

So I watch him carefully for the subtle signs that things are not right: his becoming cranky when playing, his coat taking a turn for the worse, a loss of appetite, or using soft surfaces like bedding, clothing, or towels as a toilet. I use pH strips to monitor the acid-alkaline balance of his urine on a regular basis and have become masterful at catching urine samples to take into the vet at the merest hint of trouble. I've also learned that once a litter box is soiled (especially with feces) he will not use it until it is cleaned. We need six litter boxes in the house to encourage good toilet habits. Recently, he decided that using a box that cleans itself is his best toilet ever.

Reiki plays two important roles in helping him with this condition: first, it is a way of monitoring. Sometimes his request for Reiki is the first sign of trouble. When he isn't feeling well, he will lie on his back and spread his back legs, directing me to put my hands over his lower abdomen. When that is no longer an issue and I try to put my hands in this area, he gives me a look as if to say,

47

"Back off, that's private!" And second, when he is having problems, Reiki effectively manages his pain.

Recurrent urinary tract problems aren't Blessing's only challenge. He has anatomical anomalies that require attention as well. Along with a misshapen pelvis, he has two extra vertebrae in his spine and one extra rib. They all give him the shape of a football player with a massive head and shoulders flowing into tapered hips. This makes him an excellent climber as he is able to use his front legs to propel himself up vertical surfaces. If he lived in the mountains, I'm sure he'd be rock climbing. Last but not least, he has an unusual gait. These idiosyncrasies of his bone structure mean that he needs continued chiropractic adjustments.

Initially, he saw a veterinary chiropractor who used an instrument called an activator; it ensures precise targeting of the area but makes a loud click every time it is used. Because of his fear of loud noises, Blessing would freeze, making it difficult for an adjustment to stay in place. Now he receives manual adjustments only and has been more accepting of them because they don't make a loud noise.

He was introduced to Cranial Sacral Therapy, a gentle form of touch which releases tension and energy blocks in the head and spine to allow the free flow of cerebrospinal fluid. It is very useful for chronic pain. This is a therapeutic modality he adores, so his veterinarian uses it in between each chiropractic adjustment, and he just purrs. He has become so relaxed with her that she is able to work with his badly-damaged face and jaw.

I found that his Count Dracula look - a pronounced overbite complete with two fangs hanging out over his closed mouth - was due to a strong kick to the lower jaw, estimated to have occurred a year before I rescued him. This kick left him with vertical fractures of the upper and lower jaws and a temporomandibular joint (which connects the lower jaw or mandible to the scull) that goes out of whack. Once, when I talked with him via an animal communicator, I got an image of Blessing spraying against a refrigerator and a man's boot kicking his jaw to get him out of the way. The legacy of this kick is recurring pain which has been dramatically reduced by a homeopathic remedy. Still, he isn't shy about letting me know when he needs help.

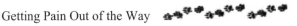

From the extensive nature of our Reiki sessions, Blessing and I are deeply bonded at an energetic level. This bond plays out in two ways. First, he can send me signals I receive within my body. For example, when there are changes in air pressure with an oncoming storm, he gets a strong headache. I then pick up a sensation in the right side of my face by the temporomandibular joint, as if someone hit me really hard. On his most difficult days, the pain will go from that joint up into my forehead and give me a headache. There are even times when things get really bad and his tongue hangs out of his mouth because he cannot quite keep it closed. It doesn't take a mental giant to figure out that he is in pain. Any of these signals tell me that he needs Reiki immediately. The second aspect of our energetic bond is that he is capable of blocking, diverting all my self-treatments and *distance* sessions for his own use when he needs them, as I described in Chapter Three.

And then there are the days when he feels great and his mischievous side shines. He becomes cocky and wants to play. My considerably older cat, Friend, is seldom in the mood to indulge him. But that doesn't stop him from trying. One day he was perched, waiting to pounce. Friend was grumpy because her back was out of alignment and she was waiting to see the veterinary chiropractor the next day. As she walked by him, he jumped her and the force of it adjusted her spine. If his jumps could be consistently precise and delivered only on an as-required basis, I could save a pile of money on veterinary bills.

If he persists in bothering her, Friend will usually punch him in the jaw. Why he doesn't avoid activating her strong right hook is beyond me. You'd think his jaw pain would keep him in line, but nothing could be further from the truth. Somehow, his urge to pounce on her overtakes any common sense.

Mostly he bugs my other cat, Kahlua, who is closer in age and thus more likely to indulge him. They start to play chase and he becomes over-excited. Then he plays rough. She screams and I take him to another room for a time-out. His cocky self-assurance disappears in an instant. His tail drags and he looks sad. He is hypersensitive to censure and yet has no sense of limits. Once the time-out is over, he forgets about the incident altogether and resorts

to mischief again. Obviously, this active, playful side demands expression.

His emotional volatility shows up when he goes outdoors on his harness, an adventure he has come to enjoy. He loves to explore, as long as the area is bounded by bushes and fencing. But put him in a open area and he goes wild. His pupils widen, he pulls at his leash, and he growls so fiercely that I have to put him in his kennel until he settles down. This behavior happens repeatedly when he is exposed to uninterrupted vistas or when he hears an unexpected, loud noise. His behavior reminds me of Post-Traumatic Stress Disorder, a malady in which those who have been severely traumatized re-visit the traumatic situation when triggered by a sensory cue. As a result, Blessing needs continued, intensive Reiki for his emotional issues.

Some people see Blessing as a very wounded cat with deep scars on many levels of his being. Yet he has made enormous progress in his return to wholeness. I note the changes in our five years together: from a cat whose eyes were sad and deadened, to ones that glisten with impishness and life; from a cat whose tail dragged as he slunk around fearfully, to a fluffy banner held high with pride; from a cat who cowered, to one who is the master of his castle. Working with him has been deeply satisfying.

Blessing is high-maintenance; he continues to need extensive Reiki supported by varieties of other care. And from time to time, he tests the unconditional nature of my love for him by refusing to use the litter box. Still, we are a unit bonded by Reiki and worth every bit of patience, trust, and time we can give each other. Besides, I have a thing for dark brown fur that is long and silky, for that long bushy tail, for that benign Count Dracula look. He has captured my heart and I am more deeply in love than ever.

Through Reiki, I've been able to make a positive difference for pets in pain. Cheekie needed pain management but could not receive medication. Crackle was in the kind of discomfort many pregnant moms will identify with, one that could only be alleviated through birthing. And Blessing will rely on Reiki for life as his body goes awry. These pets have taught me of Reiki's important role in easing levels of physical and emotional pain that range from mild discomfort to excruciating, over the short- and long-term. In such instances, Reiki can help make life worth living.

They have also taught me how sharing Reiki reduces my sense of helplessness in the face of pain and suffering. Through Reiki, I can be there for them and with them. It reminds me that in times of great distress, I have something to offer. I can be of service. And even though my contribution is a minor one, I do it with care and precision, not only to lift the spirits of those I am serving and those who surround them, but as importantly, to lift me out of my own problem space with an act of giving to others.

Chapter 6

Nourishing Emotional Health:

Lessons in Limitation

Pets feel emotions including love, hate, anger, fear, jealousy, sadness, and joy. Like us, they can become anxious and even depressed. Yet, while we have emotions in common with our cats and dogs, each species expresses them differently. For example, while we may shrink away from something we fear, cats may hiss, and dogs may bite. When they urinate on the floor instead of in the litter box, pick fights with members of the household, begin to lick compulsively, or withdraw into a closet, we know that something is wrong. Using Reiki to address this wrong is the focus of this chapter.

The stories in this chapter feature five cats: Sammy, Muggins, Buffalo Bill, Geoffrey, and Mouser. By focusing on cats, I am not suggesting that dogs are problem-free. They can suffer emotional problems like separation anxiety, fear biting, or submissive urination. But since cats and dogs are distinct species, they react differently to the same situation. Take tail wagging. See that on a dog and you know he is friendly. See that on a cat and you know he is vexed. So for the sake of clarity and cohesion, I've chosen to devote this chapter to cats whose emotions and behaviors are often misunderstood, although the underlying lessons I've learned apply to their canine counterparts as well.

The underlying theme in this chapter is about limitation. These limitations include difficulties with the human-pet bond because the pet's person cannot understand what the pet is trying to communicate. They also encompass the constraints of genetics, temperament, and household situation that impede the pet's

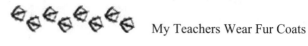

journey to wellness. And they include the frustrations and handicaps I deal with, as a Reiki practitioner trying to help pets with emotional problems.

Many people find it difficult to understand emotional problems in cats. Some may resort to punishment to keep a cat thought of as spiteful, in line. Others may take a tough love approach and let cats who are emotional basket cases fend for themselves. What many people fail to understand is that these situations may call for veterinary care.

Often, what looks like a behavioral problem is really medically-based, whether it is housesoiling, fighting, or over-grooming. For example, cats who urinate outside their litter boxes may have painful crystals in their urine, a potentially lethal situation for males. An older pet who suddenly picks fights may have a hormonal imbalance like hyperthyroidism. Parasites may irritate a pet's skin so much that he licks himself bald. Rather than risking the life of a pet who needs urgent medical attention or sharing Reiki with parasites and bacteria to help them thrive, my first question to the pet's person is, "Has your pet been examined by a veterinarian?" When the veterinarian says the pet is healthy, the problem may revert back to me. Such problems have varying causes.

Sometimes, genetics and early history influence a pet in ways that make her difficult to live with, as they did with a very shy cat I call Muggins and a bully I named Buffalo Bill. Human ignorance may be the root cause of some pets' problems, because the people in their households have inadvertently created conditions that drive them up the wall. Cats I named Buffalo Bill, Mouser, and Geoffrey fit into this category. And sometimes the behavioral diagnosis is used when a veterinarian is stumped, as happened to a cat I named Sammy.

Sammy was a young cat whose long, elegant tail had been amputated after being caught in an elevator door. The operation was successful; the outcome was not. He started to gnaw the end of his tail. Another inch of the tail was removed. It healed; he

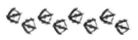

continued to barber it. Various medications were tried without success. With all that Sammy had been through, he was becoming anxious and needy.

Having exhausted the conventional veterinary repertoire, his people consulted a cat behaviorist. She listened to his history, looked at the bald stripe along what was left of his tail, and then called me in for an energetic assessment because she believed he was experiencing phantom pain.

I ran my hand along his body about an inch above his fur. The fur rose as my hand neared the base of his tail. I continued to feel a thickness well beyond the existing tail tip, as if I was in contact with a phantom tail. We reasoned that Sammy was aware of this energy blockage and was trying to remove it with his tongue. We concluded that he didn't have a behavioral problem, he had an energetic one; so we recommended a month of Reiki.

We started with three, one-hour sessions spaced closely together, and then went to weekly visits. After his first Reiki session, Sammy showed no interest in his tail for almost a week; and after five sessions, he had turned over a new leaf. My time with Sammy had been short and sweet, proving that sometimes miracles do happen and such stories have a happy ending.

If we go beyond a case such as Sammy's, whose solution was relatively simple once it was accurately diagnosed, we come to the realm of obstacles and drawbacks, as cats with genetic or temperamental handicaps try to cope in their households. Take Muggins, for example.

Muggins was a very timid cat who had spent most of her two-year life under the bed. Having no history of trauma, she was shy and withdrawn by nature, an animal who found a busy household with young children more than she could bear. Her person wanted to see if Reiki could help her become more confident and social.

I sat on the floor, talking to Muggins in soft tones and sending her *distance*, and after our first session she came out from under the bed. We had five sessions in the first two weeks, supported by *distance* in between. Then we met weekly. It took a month for her

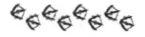

to be comfortable enough to sit beside me. Three weeks later she was confidently walking into the living room to join me for Reiki. In all, we worked together for three months.

If her person had the interest in and patience to learn Reiki, I think that Muggins would have slowly blossomed to become a more social cat. But it was not to be. Her person wanted a low-maintenance, friendly pet. She expected Reiki to change her cat's basic personality. In other words, the gap between her person's expectations of who Muggins should become and who Muggins was, was too large to bridge. Psychologists would say that they hadn't bonded. Whatever the reason, her person was disappointed that Muggins did not turn out to be the cat she would have liked for a companion, and so she stopped the sessions.

In my view, Muggins was a perfectly fine cat who was shy. And in the right household, she would thrive. In the ideal world, Muggins and her person would forge a strong bond or Muggins would find a loving home in which she could be appreciated for herself. But Muggins was in a household where she wasn't loved for being herself.

I cannot expect every person to deeply bond with the cat in her household, because love and bonding are neither rational nor predictable. Still, it frustrates me when I have so little control over such outcomes because I resonate with the cat's misery. I believe that Reiki is a wonderful modality capable of creating miracles. And sometimes, when miracles don't happen, I take it as a crushing defeat of something that is dear to me and which I greatly esteem. In other words, I come face to face with my own limitations. It's at times like these, when my ego gets in the way of accepting Reiki as it is, that I learn a hard lesson. One of those lessons came in the form of Buffalo Bill.

Buffalo Bill was a rangy cat with a very short temper. His person was proud of her cat's disagreeable temperament, taking it as a compliment that the two of them and only the two of them, could get along. Unlike Muggins and her person, Buffalo Bill and his person were strongly bonded. Then his person fell in love.

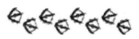

Next thing he knew, Buffalo Bill was settling into a new home with a male human and his two cats and two dogs. Seeing no need to change his ways, Buffalo Bill began to terrorize them all. His person asked his veterinarian to declaw the paws of all the cats in the household, to reduce the bleeding from the many fights that were occurring. The veterinarian strongly recommended a behavioral consultation, instead.

The behaviorist recommended some important changes. Buffalo Bill was confined to a comfortable room complete with food and litter box. At some times of the day, the rest of the pets were out and about. At others, they were kept in locked rooms, allowing Buffalo Bill the use of the house. Now, everyone could relax without fear of being attacked by the bully or having to break up fights. To help him calm down, Buffalo Bill was given medication. There were limits to how strong the doses could be and while the drug made a difference, it still didn't make him the nicest pussycat on the block. That's when I was called in to see what Reiki could do.

I hoped to use Reiki as a form of counter-conditioning, to help the cat relax in surroundings that usually made him uptight. This would require daily sessions at first. But his person would only agree to weekly visits, and those were not enough. It was like trying to get rid of an intense headache by dosing with a half a tablet of aspirin, expecting far too much from far too little. Mindful that financial issues might get in the way of helping Buffalo Bill, I tried to get his people interested in learning Reiki so they could deliver it on a more consistent and frequent basis, at less cost. Alas, they refused because they saw such little change. And after four months, the sessions were stopped.

While I believe that the lack of change was due to too little Reiki, who am I to say what Reiki should have done? It's hard in a situation like this one not to expect Reiki to deliver what I want, rather than accepting that Reiki did what it could do in less than optimal circumstances. Moreover, there is another dynamic that influenced the situation.

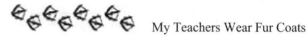

Although Buffalo Bill's person loved him deeply, she was heavily invested in their relationship as it was. She was his person, the only one with whom he could be gentle. She saw herself as valiant and brave - someone who put up with a cat so dangerous that no one else would want him. She was not impressed when he started to warm to me. All I could do was watch envy unfold and shudder.

If he slowly became more like a regular pussycat, what would have happened to her image as his savior? At some level, it was easier to keep him separated and heavily drugged than to face up to her investment in the status quo. And when I think like that, I'm aware of how judgmental I can be.

I believe in doing everything possible to help a pet. I have little tolerance for situations in which that does not happen and I become dissatisfied. Part of me continues to judge his person as deficient and part of me wonders what I could have done differently, to help his person accept the idea of change. And when I think like that, I realize my own handicap, for I am far better at working with pets than I am with people.

Yet, with some pets and their people, there is no problem in my establishing rapport. This is usually the case because the person is bonded and very committed to the pet, and sees me as a help rather than a hindrance in reaching the goal of pet wellness. Such was the case with Geoffrey and his person.

My heart went out to Geoffrey when we met, for I'd never seen a more miserable looking animal. His eyes were sad and he carried himself with resignation, as if to say that his life was not worth living. Of course, to him it wasn't. He was on anti-anxiety medication. For the past six months, he'd been wearing an Elizabethan collar (a cone around his neck that prevented him from grooming himself). That cone interfered with his ability to eat and drink, so he would often spill his kibble or accidentally splash himself with water. Because of that, the air wouldn't waft through his whiskers and he couldn't get the necessary feedback to easily go through doors or accurately land on shelves or

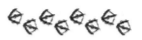

counters. Most of his family members did not respect him, calling him a dumb cat because of his problems. They did not value his privacy, thinking nothing of waking him up with a loud noise or a poke when he was in a deep sleep. His only sources of solace were the one person to whom he was bonded and the family dog. His only pleasure in life was to watch the birds come to the feeder by the window.

Unable to handle living in a loud and noisy household, filled with the blaring sounds of television and family fights, he had resorted to self-mutilation - systematically barbering his fur to bare skin and then starting to lick it raw. This over-grooming gave him peace. Grooming is a natural behavior that not only keeps a cat's coat clean, but also relaxes him by releasing endorphins (natural painkillers) in the brain. You might notice that anytime a cat is embarrassed (for example by missing a shelf he wanted to jump to), he will start to groom. When stressed, the urge to groom increases because of its soothing nature; but over-grooming has a painful cost: it's like having an itch that you scratch because it gives you relief, only to find it become more itchy so you scratch it again. In this way, Geoffrey was on a never-ending treadmill of non-stop grooming under stress.

When allergies and parasites were ruled out as probable causes of the cat's self-mutilation, the veterinarian suggested the problem was behavioral. And Geoffrey needed more than anti-anxiety drugs. Things had to change in his household as well.

A behaviorist made a number of recommendations which his person followed. She put a tall cat tree in the kitchen window so he could watch the birds at an anxiety-reducing height. And she made it the one, out-of-bounds area in the house. The new rule was that when Geoffrey was in his tree, he was not to be disturbed under any circumstances. Instead of the Elizabethan cone, she bought a special collar that looks like the kind people wear for whiplash. This allowed Geoffrey access to his face, while still making it impossible for him to groom his body. With his new collar, eating and drinking became much easier, and he got feedback from his whiskers so he could explore his environment and jump on things. Every day, his person removed his collar for short periods to allow the air to circulate on his neck. At such times, he was closely supervised so he would not re-start the cycle of over-grooming.

Geoffrey was fortunate because his person stepped up to the plate and showed her commitment to helping him get well, by making the changes the behaviorist suggested. And then she implemented the most extensive of those recommendations, hiring a Reiki practitioner. I say extensive because some pets require a great deal of time with Reiki to manifest lasting results; this is often the case with those who self-mutilate. In such cases, it is helpful if the client agrees to daily visits for the first four or five days, then cutting back to every second day, and further reducing the frequency of the sessions based on the pet's reaction. The pet's person needs to be willing to commit the resources for what may seem to be slow progress, at first; but not everyone is convinced of Reiki's merit or chooses to afford this option. Geoffrey was one of the lucky ones, for his person was ready to commit to Reiki if it would help him, and she carefully set money aside to pay for it. Because of her, Geoffrey and I had enough time to allow Reiki to truly facilitate his healing - over a year.

We started Reiki with four daily sessions in a row, followed by twice weekly sessions and, over the course of a year, reduced them to once a week. Some days he wanted *distance* and others, *hands on.* When he would permit *hands on,* I'd use a symbol I was taught in Level Two Reiki to help with mental and emotional issues. Then I'd place my hands on him and he would release whatever emotion he was feeling that day, such as anger, fear, or grief. Geoffrey would communicate his feeling state to me; it would travel up my arm to the part of my body where I'd normally feel that particular emotion, and then I'd feel its release through my heart. I wasn't doing the releasing on Geoffrey's behalf. Rather, he was communicating his method of releasing with me, since I pick up sensations with my body.

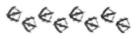

Slowly, Geoffrey started to relax. His healing journey from self-mutilation was marked by segments of progress followed by setback. Gradually, the periods of progress increased and those of setback, decreased until they disappeared. And I'm delighted that Geoffrey no longer self-mutilates.

It took more than Reiki to help Geoffrey. The modifications in the household went some way to help him. Slowly, he was weaned off his medication and let go of his special collar. And as long as his person is mindful of household dynamics and provides him with Reiki during stressful times, he should be fine.

I hold Geoffrey and his person as a model cat-person pair, committed to his healing. And I wouldn't hesitate to make time for them should it become necessary, because I believe we are all working toward the same goal. I tend to take it for granted that the pet's person would want what is best for her pet, enabling me to focus exclusively on that pet. But that isn't always the nature of the situation I face.

So, I have a choice. I can either limit myself to dealing only with pets whose people are positive and cooperative about Reiki and about helping their pets get well, or I can work to transcend my limitations. Some of the pets with whom I have shared Reiki, have exhorted me to push myself beyond my level of comfort with people. Instead of restricting my focus to Reiki and enhancing the pet's receptivity to it, they are telling me that I need to expand it - to help the pet's person become more receptive to the pet having Reiki.

I cannot force someone to arrange for Reiki for their pet. And I cannot force someone to continue with Reiki sessions. My challenge is to find solutions to household situations in a way that more actively and positively includes the pet's person, as well as the pet. When I have risen to this challenge, the solution can be quite different from what I had imagined. Mouser's case is an example.

Mouser was a middle-aged, male Oriental shorthair who supervised an all-female harem of four cats, one dog, and a

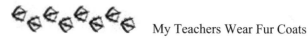

human. His person provided the cats with a large fish tank and a big-screen TV tuned to animal programs. They were allowed to sit on all the soft furniture and there was no shortage of toys. But something was wrong with Mouser.

Every time someone came to the door, Mouser went ballistic. He would hover by the entrance and start to caterwaul, saving his most vocal performances for men. He'd likely had little experience of them when he was a young kitten, and cats need such exposure between the ages of two and seven weeks, to be comfortable. Other than that, Mouser was fine.

For years, his behavior problem was ignored because it erupted infrequently, for what few visitors the household had, were largely female; and Mouser was fine with them.

One day, a water pipe burst and extensive plumbing repairs were needed. The plumber made several trips in and out of the house to get parts and supplies from his truck. With each successive re-entry, Mouser became more agitated. His operatic range increased as he let forth an aria so shrill that it would take the enamel off your teeth. And then he attacked the plumber. When they were able to be separated, the bleeding and bruised plumber left the scene, never to return.

Mouser's person knew that something had to be done, so she consulted a behaviorist who noted that the household was anxiety-ridden. His person was so anxious about her pets' safety that the cats had been declawed, in the hope that they would be less inclined to jump, even though Oriental shorthairs love to rest in high places; cat trees had been removed and all high shelves were crowded with ornaments to prevent the cats from using them; and they were confined indoors, again because of fears for their safety. No wonder Mouser was uptight.

One of the behaviorist's recommendations was for more interactive play to simulate predation and reduce his anxiety levels. Cats are predators by nature and since they have been so recently domesticated, there is still a lot of wild in every cat. A wild cat hunts several times a day: watching for prey, stalking,

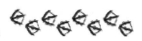

then pouncing and, from time to time, catching, killing, and eating them. Without the opportunity to exercise this behavioral repertoire, the cat's arousal level increases. Blocked from expression, it slowly builds to a point from which it is difficult to reverse, where even the smallest stimulus - like the rustle of a piece of paper - sets the cat off.

At that point, veterinarians and behaviorists usually recommend that the cat be given medication for a period of time to lower the arousal level, and ask the cat's person to change things in the environment so that the situation can be brought under control. In Mouser's case, this would include offering him outdoor experience (through a cat enclosure or the use of a cat fence to keep him safely in the backyard), daily interactive play sessions, and the availability of different levels of height, so that all the cats in the household could arrange themselves in a way that would lessen their overall anxiety.

Mouser's person refused to implement these recommendations. She wouldn't consider medication because she believed it meant her cat was crazy. The cat was not mentally ill by any means, just going crazy from the rules of an anxiety-driven household. The idea of cat trees was nixed. And she wasn't ready to think about any outdoor experience. At that point, the behaviorist suggested re-homing Mouser, but she wasn't willing to let him go. And even if she was, who would be willing to take a troubled cat? There was one more option to try: Reiki.

I came to our first session with the behaviorist in tow, since Mouser's person was always anxious about strangers coming to the house. The cat ignored the behaviorist, but I was a different matter. He was not impressed by the dogs' scents on my clothes from two previous clients of the day. One sniff and he started to howl. Then he retreated under a nearby table to keep watch on me, interrupted by sporadic bursts of caterwauling.

I stayed in the front hall and squatted, sending *distance* to him with cupped hands. Suddenly, he stopped singing, came over to my hands, and opened his mouth to taste the odor (known as the

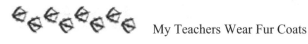

Flehmen response). But there was nothing between my hands but a ball of energy. With a puzzled look on his face, he retreated back under the table. He repeated these actions several times. When he stayed in one spot for five minutes, I figured it was okay to come into the house. So I went and sat on a recliner, all the time continuing *distance* to him through cupped hands. Twenty minutes later, Mouser came over, jumped on the top of the recliner and sprawled, quietly purring.

Based on this performance, his person was ready to accept the idea that Reiki might help him. And she was willing to allow frequent sessions. We started with a daily, one-hour session for four days, followed by visits two and three times a week, and over the course of several months, reduced those to once a week. Mouser improved with almost every session, and there was an added benefit as well: other members of the household, including his person, hitchhiked on the Reiki that was filling up the room and became more relaxed and settled. After several sessions, his person became interested enough to learn Reiki herself.

In time, she became more confident in having people over and her friends remarked at how much calmer Mouser seemed. By learning and sharing Reiki, she reduced her own anxiety levels, as well as those of her furry companions. But it took even longer before she was able to take bigger steps for the cats' benefit. Three years later, she was ready to consider an outdoor enclosure. I don't think she ever bought a cat tree. Regardless, Mouser still did well. And he taught me a valuable lesson about how to transcend what appears to be a limited situation, by looking for a broader solution.

The pets in this chapter have taught me that while emotional problems run the gamut, Reiki may be one element in their solution. They have enabled me to have a clearer understanding of the powerful influence that can be exerted by the pet's person, not only over the pet, but also over me. Most of the time, that person lets the pet and I share Reiki, relatively unfettered. With Sammy and Geoffrey, the circumstances aligned so beautifully

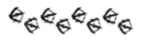

that I could focus solely on sharing Reiki with them. But there are times when the pet's person thwarts the Reiki process, warning me that I cannot take such a person for granted.

Both Muggins and Buffalo Bill have taught me that when the pet's person cannot accommodate to the pet, either as she is or is becoming through Reiki, then its role in the broader context of the pet's household appears to be negligible, regardless of the results it facilitates. And they have led me to search for more appropriate solutions. In such cases, I feel the need to enhance the person's receptivity to Reiki for her pet. When I cannot do so, or choose not to, sessions may be subverted or terminated as the pet's person lets his own agenda unfold. Then I am smack up against my limitations: I have failed.

Why can't I find a magic formula that will enable Reiki to succeed on my terms, resolving any problem so that the pet is better off from my point of view? Largely because that is not the purpose of Reiki. Reiki does whatever needs to be done, going wherever it needs to go. I must face the limits of my appreciation of what Reiki is, when it crushes my ego in the process by making me look like we have failed. For Reiki does not exist to make me look good and I am not perfect. Rather than looking for perfection, I need to embrace my limitations, knowing that my role may be smaller than I sometimes wish and the outcomes different from what I would have wanted.

Sometimes when I rise to the occasion, an elegant solution awaits both the pet, like Mouser, and the overall circumstances in which he finds himself. And when such a problem is resolved, I realize that what might look like an obstacle within the pet or his household, may actually be an opportunity. And it is up to me to make the most of the opportunities that present themselves, knowing full well that I cannot always rise above my limitations.

Chapter 7

Coping with Cancer: Lessons in Compassion

Dealing with cancer can be an exercise in suffering for both the person and his pet, because for many of us, a diagnosis of cancer equates with calamity. Fear of loss, worries about pain, and financial pressures are some of the elements of misery that contribute to our ordeal. When a beloved pet is involved, the situation becomes more complex as we try to decode his wishes, reactions, and progress. In this chapter, I share stories of pets with cancer, showing how Reiki offered comfort, helped them manage their pain, enhanced their recovery from surgery or chemotherapy, or acted as a palliative in the absence of treatment. Most especially for pets with cancer, the simple act of sharing Reiki buffers their suffering with compassion. And so in this chapter, I share what I have learned about the facets of compassion from the pets who brought them to my attention. Before I describe some of the pets and their circumstances, I want to return to the general challenges before the person and his pet.

The human partner strongly influences how the quantity and quality of his pet's life is balanced. If the cancer is treatable, the human has to decide which options to take: surgery to remove the tumor if there is one, radiation to destroy cancerous tissue with radioactive isotopes, and/or chemotherapy to slow down the growth of cancer with chemicals. The objective remains the same regardless of the options selected: to give his pet an added lease on life in relative comfort, minimizing often incredible intensities of pain and protecting her from infection due to a compromised immune system. Even providing enough food is fettered with obstacles, for the side effects of many treatments - nausea, vomiting, diarrhea, and anorexia - make eating the last thing on her mind.

Facing this situation, the person may project his own fears about cancer onto his pet, who then adds this to a growing bank of anxiety building up from the invasive nature of some of the treatments. She may become depressed when amputation and lack of energy limit what she can now do. As her illness progresses, the emotional

temperature of the household can change, for there may be family arguments about financial priorities if expensive treatments are involved. To make matters worse, her animal companions may now shun her, responding to ancient wisdom that associating with the weak threatens one's own survival. These are some of the aspects of suffering, and it is the context within which people whose pets have cancer seek holistic therapies like Reiki.

The first pet in this chapter is Spiffy, a dog whose person brings out the shadow side of my compassion by putting me in the seat of judgment.

I temper my feelings about what happened to Spiffy, by describing the success of interventions with Victoria, a dog with a benign rectal tumor. Then it is Janvier's turn to show how a feline gift continues to help me understand compassion at a deep, physical level. His lesson sets the stage for my work with Samantha, a dog undergoing surgery and chemotherapy for cancer of the jaw. And finally, I introduce Timmy, a cat who has helped me build on Janvier's lesson to the point that we can share all the facets of compassion together. Let's begin with Spiffy.

Spiffy was an elderly, feisty dog with cancer in one leg. His person was repulsed by the idea of amputation despite veterinary advice to proceed with it, and allowed only radiation instead. I was called to supplement his person's Reiki sessions with him. Already, I was less than impressed that his person could make such a decision, for I would have proceeded with amputation. Little did I realize that Spiffy's situation, needing a surgery which his person couldn't abide, would make me confront how easily I judge rather than accept that which I cannot change.

After his radiation treatments were completed, we watched Spiffy become stronger, gradually being able to bear weight on his leg. However, he had to wear an Elizabethan collar, a cone wrapped around his head to prevent him from chewing at the tumor site. In short order, the tumor started to grow again, making the area look worse and worse. His person was now ready to accept the need for surgery because he couldn't tolerate the appearance of the lesion on his handsome dog. I wasn't concerned that his person's decision was

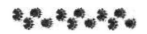

the right one; I was worried that it came too late. With surgery, most, but not all, of the tumor was able to be removed.

We supported Spiffy with extensive amounts of Reiki. I sent *distance* to him during surgery; immediately after, I started *hands on* for two hours, leaving his person to continue with Reiki for several more. That night, I sent him two *distance* sessions of one hour each, adding to the Reiki he received through his person.

The next evening Spiffy was home, greeting me at the door, barking, and wagging his tail. The only way I could tell that he'd had surgery was by the splint on his leg. Reiki had helped a speedy recovery and his wounds soon healed completely. Unfortunately, because the entire tumor could not be removed, it metastasized and he died three months later.

It saddens me when I know that Spiffy could have lived much longer if the tumor had been removed in the first place, and I had to come to terms with the fact that it was not my decision to make. Over the years, I've learned that caregiver decisions are not easy because you need to integrate what is best for your pet with what you can tolerate. Yet, I am always tempted to judge. I have a way to go before I am fully able to extend compassion to all human caregivers, regardless of the actions they take - having faith that they acted as best they could, even if their actions do not make sense to me. And at those times, when I despair of the shortsightedness that seems to come with the human condition, I focus on situations where the word, tumor, doesn't mean that death is imminent. Such was the case with Victoria.

Victoria was a senior American Cocker Spaniel who had surgery to remove a benign rectal tumor. A few months later, it grew back; this time, it was inoperable. Poor Victoria started to bleed from the rectum, sometimes a little and sometimes a lot.

Her treatment had three parts: medication to prevent tumor cells from being replicated, psyllium added into her food so she could more easily pass her stools, and about six hours of Reiki daily. When she wanted *hands on*, I'd work on her lower back, the base of her tail, and the area between her abdomen and pelvis. Mostly, she preferred *distance*. The bleeding stopped.

Curious about the effect of Reiki, her person (a health care professional) had the sessions cut back. The bleeding started again. Reiki was resumed and the bleeding stopped again. And so we continued with Reiki. At the same time, her medication was permanently discontinued.

When I worked with Victoria, I felt her tumor in my body. But after working with her for about two years, I told her person that I couldn't sense the tumor any more. Her veterinarian found that the tumor had shrunk. Now it was able to be removed completely and so she proceeded with surgery. From that time on, Victoria was never bothered by rectal bleeding again.

The feeling of her tumor in my body is a type of experience I have at times, with pets who share the state of their physical and emotional selves with me. And I will never forget the first time it happened, with a cat called Janvier.

Janvier was a cat who needed love and attention, but whose body was covered with open tumors giving off the distinct smell of rotting flesh. Usually when a cat is terminally ill and needy, members of his care team band together to provide him with emotional as well as medical support. As long as he can tolerate it, they will offer comfort by stroking his fur, giving him a cuddle or, if this is too painful, sitting beside him and talking in soft tones. In Janvier's case, many of the people on his health care team found it difficult to get near enough to him to look after routine needs, let alone spend extra time in his presence. (Fortunately, his person was not one of them.)

It did not occur to me to be repulsed by his body, for he had touched my heart and compelled me to act. To me, the situation was straightforward: he was a cat; he was sick; he needed Reiki; and he wanted *hands on*. So I visited him at the veterinary clinic, crawled into his double-wide, floor-level cage, and sat beside him delivering *hands on*, his preferred mode of Reiki. He responded with a chorus of purrs. And then something very unexpected occurred.

I was at home sending *distance* to him, when I felt bodily sensations that I knew were not mine. I felt his tumors in my body, not only in the places I knew about but in three others as well. Concerned, I called the veterinary clinic to describe what I felt; and

later that day, his veterinarian confirmed three new tumors in the exact locations I had described.

I was overwhelmed by the gift Janvier had given to me, for he introduced me to clairsentience, the ability to feel in my body what is happening to a pet. To me, it is the ultimate act of communication, for my only access to it is when the pet in question is willing to share. I will always be grateful to Janvier for his generosity. Thanks to him, I can help pets in ways that would otherwise not be possible, by understanding the physical nature of the suffering they bear.

Janvier's gift helped one of my canine clients, Samantha. She was a large breed dog in the prime of life when she got cancer of the jaw. If she went untreated, she would live another few months; with surgery and chemotherapy she would likely enjoy another 18. Faced with these options and the optimism of her veterinarian, who believed that the dog's large size would enable her to handle the treatment well, Samantha had the surgery. Her people contacted me to do what I could, to reduce the side-effects of the treatment - pain and nausea.

My first task was to help her recover from surgery. Needless to say, her mouth was very sore, so I gave her *hands on* on the side of her mouth and neck. She kept my hands glued to the area for one and a half hours; I felt extremely hot sensations in my hands. I've noticed that when a pet needs a massive dose of Reiki in short order, I feel intense heat in my hands and body. It is important to stay grounded when this size of draw is channeling through or I become dizzy. Since this tells me that the pet badly needs what I'm helping her to get, I try to hang in as long as possible. I supplemented Samantha's *hands on* sessions with *distance*. For the first two weeks following her surgery, I saw her daily and then my visits decreased to three times a week, until she was ready for chemotherapy.

One afternoon Janvier's gift re-surfaced. I was in a coffee shop sipping a drink and sending a *distance* to Samantha when I got a vile taste in my mouth. In spite of trying popcorn, mouthwash, and many other things, the taste stayed with me for four hours. I asked Samantha's person what might have been happening with the dog at the time that *distance* was sent. Apparently, that particular *distance* session had coincided with a hydrogen peroxide rinse, one of four

71

daily rinses given to keep her mouth free of infection. From that time on, I got her feeding schedule so I could avoid the awful taste. And to help Samantha, her people decided to delay the rinse for 40 minutes after she had eaten, to allow her to enjoy her meal before it was washed down with the vile-tasting but necessary liquid. All of this is thanks to Janvier.

Samantha continued with about an hour of *hands on* three times a week, until her first chemotherapy session. She was injected in the veterinary clinic early in the morning. When I was allowed to see her in the late afternoon, she was lying in her cage, shaking and unable to retain food or water. I gave her a two-hour, full-body, *hands on* session and then sent her *distance* that night. She left the clinic the next morning.

For the next seven days, I did two-hour, *hands on* sessions with her everyday. At each session, Samantha insisted that I keep my hands over her liver and kidneys most of time. She instinctively seemed to protect these organs from the damage that chemotherapy could do to them.

Meanwhile, I learned from my Reiki Master of the time, that it was important to start Reiki when the chemotherapy starts. So when the time came for her next chemotherapy treatment, I did *distance* for one hour when she received the injection in the morning, followed by two hours when I could. When I went to see her in the late afternoon, she was standing up and alert, able to eat, drink, and toilet. The staff were very surprised because they'd never seen a dog respond so positively to chemotherapy before. Again, I gave her a full-body *hands on* session followed by *distance* in the evening, and then seven days in a row of intense, two-hour *hands on* sessions.

While she was initially expected to undergo five chemotherapy treatments, her veterinarian was satisfied enough with her progress to stop after the third. And much to his surprise, the expected damage to her liver and kidneys was not found. Samantha surpassed the optimistic prognosis of 18 months by a country mile. Three years after our sessions had ended, she was alive and well.

There have also been good news stories about feline cancer clients, the best example of which is Timmy, an orange and white cat with a sense of humor. At age twelve, he was diagnosed with

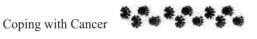

inflammatory bowel disease and treated with medication. But he continued to vomit, have diarrhea, and lose weight, so he underwent exploratory surgery. The veterinarian took biopsies and inserted a feeding tube through which he could be force fed. From the biopsies, Timmy was diagnosed with alimentary lymphosarcoma, a common form of cancer that affects the stomach, intestines, liver, and associated lymph nodes. He spent almost two weeks in the hospital.

He wasn't recovering from his surgery very well and showed little interest in eating on his own, so I was asked to provide Reiki. As he started to receive it, he sat up as if to ask, "What's going on?" and according to his person, immediately started to change: he decided to live. During that first session, we heard his bowels making sounds. This was cause for celebration, for we'd been told that the key to his recovery would be the restoration of his bowel function. At the end of that session, Timmy got up, ate by mouth, and did not vomit his food back up. This was real progress, all within 24 hours of his first Reiki session.

With daily Reiki, Timmy's appetite continued and he was able to hold his food down; then he started to have normal bowel movements. His feeding tube was removed and he gradually regained his weight. He continues with the medication Prednisone, a corticosteroid. Sixteen months after surgery, he started to see a holistic veterinarian (in addition to conventional care), who introduced him to regular vitamin injections. He also started taking customized, herbal, anti-cancer formulations which are adjusted depending on the bodily sensations I pick up from Timmy during our sessions. He prefers *distance* because he has so much to do: eating, bird watching, and being charming, all the while receiving the benefits of a Reiki session. Gradually, his person took over his daily Reiki needs and I started to visit him two or three times a week, unless otherwise needed.

Janvier's gift continues to manifest in my work with Timmy. From time to time, he goes through a difficult phase, when he vomits, loses his appetite and weight, tightens his face, and becomes restless - likely evidence of pain. My lower right side (mirroring his cancer site) becomes sore as well. Then three of us intensify his Reiki: myself, his person, and his feline companion. I visit him for

three, one-hour sessions a week and provide *distance* from my home on the other days. His person gives him all the *hands on* he will tolerate, plus one and half hours of *distance* and three healing attunements a day. And his feline companion, Beauty, snuggles up to him and gives him *paws on* sessions. (Beauty's Reiki skill is described in Chapter Ten.) Then he releases a build-up of energy around the lower right side of his body.

When this first happened as we worked together, I felt a ball of pain move gradually through the right side of my body and then pop out. Build-ups of energy that started as balls of fire now come in all textures, shapes, temperatures, and sizes: some feel solid, others are gooey; the jagged ones hurt so much that they brought tears to my eyes, but others are smooth; some feel hot and others feel like ice; some are small and some are huge.

Having a sense of humor, Timmy also shares cartoon-like images with me during such sessions. When this first started, I saw his back legs in my mind's eye pushing with all their might to get rid of the energetic build-up. Recently, I saw him putting on a snorkel, goggles, rain poncho, and rubber gloves up to his armpits. The release felt gooey, so I figured that he didn't want it to explode all over him. But most of the time he deals with the release after he puts on a surgical mask, rubber gloves, and a gown. Sometimes, he sprays the build-up with a fire extinguisher and I feel ice cold as if he is freezing it out; then he will take a welding torch to liquefy it and I feel it flowing out the side of my body.

While Timmy and I share this process together, I don't believe that I am doing the releasing for him through my body. If I did, I'd likely be exhausted by our sessions and experience a headache, nausea, or lightheadedness that would last for hours longer. The form of Reiki I learned is so safe for both the recipient and the transmitter, that I never fear that my client's energetic debris will back up into me. Instead, our shared symptoms mirror a process of communication by which he keeps me apprised of his situation. I feel privileged to share this level of intimacy with him, for it comes with a tremendous amount of trust and mutual respect.

During these kinds of sessions, he can have anywhere from one to eight releases so I make sure to book my time with Timmy at the

end of my day, because a release session takes between two and three hours. If I scrimp on the time because of other commitments, it makes it harder on Timmy; so I prefer to give him my undivided attention. I can also do a release session with him through *distance* from my home but again, I need to be fully present for him. He may need more follow-up sessions to ensure that the releasing is finished. Then his face relaxes, he eats, and has a long, deep sleep. This is followed by an indeterminate period during which he gains weight and returns to his playful self.

Over time, Timmy's need for support has increased. He has a dedicated team working with him: his person, his feline companion, a conventional veterinarian, a holistic veterinarian, as well as myself. His person is dedicated to providing him with Reiki every day and she is the only person from whom he will regularly accept *hands on*. When his Reiki needed to be escalated, I taught her healing attunements - shorter, more intense sessions to take the place of the six to eight hours a day that he would otherwise need. I already mentioned that when he isn't feeling well, his feline companion, Beauty, gives him *paws on* Reiki. Yet when he is feeling well, she swats him, instead. It would be extremely difficult for a practitioner to keep up with his escalating Reiki needs, without the dedication and commitment of his person and his companion.

Timmy paid me the ultimate compliment by sharing his vision of how Reiki works with his cancer: an hourglass filled with sand that is running out of it quickly. Then a dose of Reiki arrives and pushes a large amount of sand back up, not to the top but high enough to be significant. Every time the sand starts to run down again, another dose of Reiki pushes it up. To me, it suggests that Reiki slows down the progression of time, that is, Reiki alters the time frame within which the cancer operates, extending it considerably. Timmy's cancer has never gone into remission, the stage at which it can no longer be detected in the body (even though it doesn't mean that it has disappeared). Yet, I believe that Timmy knows something about how Reiki works with cancer - because the average survival time of a cat with lymphosarcoma is six to eight months after diagnosis; for Timmy it has been over four years. Because of Timmy, I've begun to comprehend the powerful beauty of Reiki in altering the temporal

dimension of this disease. In addressing cancer, Reiki, itself, is the embodiment of compassion, establishing sufficient rapport with the cancer to gently push back its invasive agenda.

Pets with cancer have shown me the palliative dimension of Reiki. Spiffy and Samantha were able to quickly rally from painful surgeries because of it. Victoria was able to forego the side-effects of a rectal tumor (its bleeding) and Samantha, most of the nasty side-effects of chemotherapy. Through Reiki, Timmy is able to play an active part in the management of his disease. By relieving the stress on their bodies from pain or the side-effects of disease or its treatment, Reiki frees the body to do what only it can: take them on a healing path

Spiffy, Victoria, Samantha, Janvier, and Timmy allowed (and in some cases, continue to allow) me to walk beside them as they followed their healing journey. As we traveled together, they taught me about the many facets of compassion - physical, emotional, intellectual, and spiritual. One of their most important teachings has been that each of these levels has a superficial side which is more about me than about them and the context in which they suffer, and a deeper side that reflects the meaning of the concept more deeply. As I walk with them, I may experience physical sensations in reaction to their situations, such as wanting to vomit or contracting my muscles; these are simply about me and my reactions. But when I experience sensations in my own body of what they are actually enduring, I understand more clearly what is implied by the word, compassion. Similarly on an emotional level, my own feelings of hopelessness or anger say something about me and my sense of uselessness or self-righteousness. I can only offer solace to pets when I become sensitive to their feelings and moods, thereby experiencing the emotional facet of compassion. Intellectually, I may let my ego get in the way by starting to judge whether or not their people's suffering is deserved. But when I comprehend the nature of one pet's suffering and get a sense that I have grasped it, I have reached that deeper level of rapport. There are times when I see the shadow side of compassion at the spiritual level, as the pet and I engage in a battle against evil forces, for cancer presents me with images of darkness and evil. Recognizing these powerful, pervasive forces for

what they are, I surrender to Reiki and get out of the way. That is why I never direct Reiki to the cancer, regardless of the form of Reiki I am using; I don't want to take the chance of enhancing it, helping it to grow. Instead, I send Reiki to the pet as a whole and let the energy deal with the body in the way it knows best.

Thanks to Janvier's gift of clairsentience, the ability to share the physical and emotional aspects of suffering at the invitation of the pet with whom I am working, we can achieve spiritual communion, a sense of fellow feeling uniting us both with the larger whole. When this happens, I know that we are in the hands of compassion: we are truly living in the spirit of Reiki.

Chapter 8

Changing the Course of Chronic Illness:

Lessons in Perseverance

Chronic illnesses such as kidney disease, diabetes, and hyperthyroidism, have no cure. By their very nature, they can take years to develop before being recognized. The human challenge in the face of such disease is consistency: to provide quality care day in and day out. This care is an act of faith, a belief that such effort will help the pet to win life extension and possibly remission, as he races against the progression of chronic illness. As this chapter shows, there is a lot that can be done to increase the pet's comfort, slow down the progress of disability, and ensure a high quality of life - if you persevere. To illustrate this point, I have chosen four cats: Penny and Friend have kidney disease; Snowball is diabetic; and Simon suffered from hyperthyroidism. In my experience, these lessons apply equally to my canine clients.

Penny is an example of a cat whose kidney disease progressed slowly and so its care requirements could increase at a sedate pace. She is a diminutive, silver tabby with a fondness for cat treats and red toys. She is the boss of a household that includes two much-younger cats, Millie and Wes, and a human. When she was 16, she started to vomit repeatedly. On the basis of blood work and urinalysis, she was diagnosed with kidney disease.

Kidney disease often creeps up on senior cats and dogs, for by the time the pet shows signs of it, about two-thirds of the kidney has been irreparably destroyed. And as the kidney deteriorates, every other bodily organ is affected. When only 15% to 20% of the kidney's tissue remains intact, the animal dies. While there is no cure, pets can live comfortably for many years if the symptoms are managed and stress loads, reduced.

I started to visit Penny twice a week and then, when her person learned Reiki, once weekly. Now, Penny gets a daily *hands on*

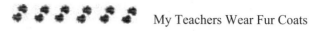

session from her person, and a once weekly healing attunement and *distance* session with me. I've learned to be careful about using healing attuncments with the frail or elderly, because agitation or aggravation of symptoms can happen with some pets who receive them. So, I make sure to always be physically present when I send the first such attunement, and stay on to monitor their reaction to it. Fortunately, Penny enjoyed them as she does all Reiki. However, she gets miffed when I am late for our meetings. On such occasions, she will snub my greeting and punctuate our session with repeated glances from the clock to me. So I prefer to meet with her on time.

Now she is 19 and the disease has progressed. So Penny receives fluids through subcutaneous hydration (that is, inserting fluids under her skin through a needle) about every two weeks. This keeps her body hydrated in spite of the large volumes of urine she releases. Otherwise, her joints and muscles would ache and her appetite would wane. She is less able to climb and jump; so cat stairs have been installed to allow her easier access to the couch and bed. And as she becomes more frail, Millie has started to challenge her leadership. Now, Penny is watchful when she crosses the living room floor, or Millie will tackle her.

As she becomes more challenged by the tasks of daily living, it is important to make Penny as comfortable as possible so she can enjoy her sunset years with confidence. The relatively gentle progression of Penny's illness meant there was time for her person to accommodate to new levels of care. But sometimes, the disease catches you unaware, and high levels of care are demanded immediately, as with my own cat, Friend.

Friend is my eldest household companion - a shorthaired, mackerel tabby cat with a red belly and under-tail that mirror her feisty personality. Her beauty equals that of Sneaky Pie Brown who, with her person Rita Mae, authors the well-known Mrs. Murphy mystery series. She joined my household as a kitten, having been found by my cat, Beakers, in an abandoned car with a bag of cat food. One day Beakers brought her home and made it clear that she was staying. And stay she did.

Friend was nine years old when, thanks to Reiki, she was diagnosed as being in the early stages of kidney disease. I thank Reiki because most times this disease isn't diagnosed until it has

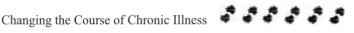

progressed much further than hers had. Reiki made early diagnosis possible.

Until then, Friend didn't much like Reiki. If I'd offer it to her, she'd indulge me in a *hands on* session for about 10 minutes while wearing a pained expression on her face, and then she'd leave. She wasn't crazy about receiving *distance* either. Then, all of a sudden she did an about-face. She started to request Reiki by chirping at me and putting her rear end near my hands when I was resting. While she looked healthy, I was alarmed at this behavioral change, especially when it continued for days.

We went to her veterinarian who agreed that Friend looked healthy. But she, too, knew that Friend's change in attitude toward Reiki meant that further investigation was warranted. Blood tests showed Friend to be in the early stages of kidney disease. Kidney function is measured in two ways, by Blood Urea Nitrogen (BUN) and creatinine levels. Friend's BUN was 9 mmol/L, well within the normal range of 3.5 to 13.0 mmol/L; her creatinine was 233 µmol/L, slightly elevated from the normal range of 88 to 177 µmol/L.

We set up a schedule for veterinary testing. Her urine is tested every two months (its specific gravity being another measure of kidney function) and her blood, every three months.

Friend started to demand at least one hour of *hands on* a day. In time, she demanded less Reiki. Eleven months after diagnosis, her kidney function values were back in the normal range (BUN was 10.7 mmol/L and creatinine, 175 µmol/L). Then, I made the mistake of reducing the amount of Reiki she received. Other clients with kidney disease had deteriorated when their daily Reiki ration was reduced, but because Friend was the first cat I knew whose values had returned to normal, I thought I could get away with less. When Friend did ask for Reiki, I was tired and often fell asleep in the middle of a session; so she really wasn't getting the extra Reiki she requested. To put it mildly, I slacked off. Suddenly, six weeks later Friend stopped eating; she was nauseated and in great pain.

X-rays showed severe gastric inflammation. That I could handle, but the blood work was a shock to both her veterinarian and myself, because her kidney function values were extremely high. Her BUN was 60 mmol/L and her creatinine, 1,861 µmol/L! Accordingly, she should have been skin and bones, totally lethargic, and foul-smelling

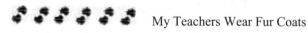

from uremia (blood poisoning). Instead, the only outward sign of her malady was a somewhat ruffled coat. She was still a pound and a half overweight, and feisty. Perhaps what Reiki she had been receiving had provided some support, but I learned the hard way that I must be diligent and consistent in my delivery of Reiki.

Friend spent a week in the hospital on intravenous fluids, and was released only when she no longer vomited her force feedings. Then, I had to keep her hydrated by giving her subcutaneous fluids daily, as well as three medications to calm her ulcerated gastrointestinal system: a stomach coater, an antacid, and a phosphorus binder. I gave her hours of *hands on* Reiki supported by friends who sent her *distance*. Over the next few days, her condition stabilized.

Two weeks later, her blood work was repeated; her BUN was 14 mmol/L and her creatinine, 286 μmol/L, results her veterinarian described as phenomenal. Sometimes, creatinine levels drop because there is muscle-wasting, but this has not been the case with Friend. So the only thing to which her results can be attributed is Reiki.

In addition, I am mindful that stress and dehydration can make it difficult for the kidneys to flush toxins from the body, leading to kidney infections. As her disease progresses, she will become more prone to such infections simply as a result of the disease itself. But for now, her kidney function values continue in the normal range. The only way her kidney disease can be detected is through the pulse-taking of Traditional Chinese Medicine. She requires her other medications (that stomach coater, antacid, and phosphorus binder) only on occasion. And her diet is a high-quality food that contains normal protein levels, rather than one specifically formulated for cats with kidney disease.

She continues to need large, regular Reiki doses to maintain her health. We worked on finding her right maintenance level: a minimum of one hour of Reiki a day except for Sundays (my day off), when she loads up with three to eight hours of *hands on* at her request. This makes Sundays a working holiday for me. *Hands on* remains her preference and when she wants it, she climbs on me and presents her hind end. If she'd like a healing attunement, she waits until I am sending one to another client and then starts to dance around and chirp. So I have a very clear idea of what she wants and

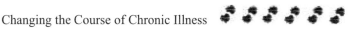

when. And when she does, I comply, sometimes feeling like I am slogging away.

I've been tempted at times to shorten our sessions and go on to other things, like laundry and shopping. But then I remind myself of the old fable about the race between Tortoise and Hare. Hare could easily win. Instead, he slacks off by taking a nap in the middle of it, because he thinks he has lots of time to beat Tortoise before the end of the course is reached. Meanwhile, Tortoise keeps steadfastly to the course, slowly and consistently making progress. Hare wakes up; and even though he is better at running, he cannot make up for lost time. And so, Tortoise wins the race.

I think of Friend being in a race where the prizes are comfort and life extension. And I am running it with her. Sometimes I am Tortoise and other times, Hare. When I am tempted to slack off on Reiki for Friend, I am like Hare. I have faith that I could call on Reiki to help her when really needed and lulled by that faith, I take the equivalent of a nap instead; I watch TV, pay my bills, vacuum, or go shopping. And then, when Friend's health gets out of hand and it is clear that she needs help fast, I pull out all the stops and provide as much Reiki as possible.

What favor is this to Friend? It condemns her to a seesaw existence, lurching from a state of reasonable health to an unnecessary health crisis. And it condemns me to emotional vacillation from the pits of guilt and despair as I witness her suffering from my neglect, to exultation when another Reiki miracle occurs. So instead, I've opted to share Reiki with the dedication and endurance of Tortoise, because I know the diligence and constancy of our Reiki sessions make Friend's life so much better.

I can appreciate how easy it is for a pet's person to slack off when her pet appears physically stable or there are competing priorities. Many times, it is as if chronic illness, itself, takes a nap, for there are periods without indicators that the illness itself is changing - for better or worse - because its progress is so slow. So anyone can be seduced by what seems to be a holding pattern. But leave it long enough and there will be a crisis. And while Reiki can help in a crisis, sometimes it is too late to turn the situation around.

I remind myself of how precious Friend is to me and how much I value having her in my life. That is how I get the strength to

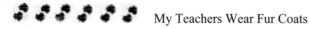

persevere when there are so many other things I think I should be doing. And when I know I'm going to falter from the overwhelm of needy clients along with my own needy pet, I call on friends to provide her with daily *distance* sessions until I can get my life back in order.

Some clients of kidney cats have taken them to veterinarians who suggest that the levels of Reiki can be reduced when alternative treatments are in place. But given my experience with Friend (who has used herbal supplements and homeopathic remedies), I wouldn't chance it. I now know that a relatively large amount of Reiki shared on a consistent basis is required to keep a cat with kidney disease well.

For pets with kidney disease, Reiki seems to be an energetic form of dialysis. Likely because the disease is one where tissue cannot regenerate, withdrawing Reiki leaves a pet only her diseased bodily resources to fall back on, and this is not enough. Even by bolstering her inner resources through Reiki, she cannot rebuild destroyed kidney tissue. So I am reminded that Reiki is palliative. It can reverse the conventional signs of disease, but take it away and they rear their ugly heads again. In this way, I have been reminded of the importance of constancy and devotion to Reiki sessions - in other words, the value of perseverance.

Diabetes is another chronic disease that can affect pets, especially if they are overweight. It occurs when the pancreas does not produce enough insulin to drive sugar out of the blood vessels to where it is needed as a source of energy. As a result, blood sugar levels rise and spill out into the urine, thereby causing urine sugar levels to rise. One of the first signs of diabetes can be increased thirst. All of a sudden, a pet who had ignored the water bowl now lives with her head hanging over it. And since what goes in does go out, the litter box often resembles a swimming pool or the dog begins to house soil. The animal may lose weight and energy level. The disease is managed by diet (often specially-prepared or prescription foods), a strict feeding regime, and the use of insulin. Such was the case with Snowball, an ivory, longhaired cat.

When she was first diagnosed, her person couldn't bear the thought of giving her insulin injections twice a day and was ready to

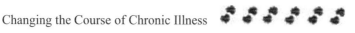

have her euthanized. But with patience and careful training by veterinary staff, she mastered the fine art of injections instead.

When I was asked to share Reiki with Snowball, I consulted a Reiki colleague who has a diabetic family member. She's found that those diabetics who receive Reiki daily on a consistent basis, need to carefully monitor their insulin levels, because they often need to be lowered. Withdraw regular Reiki sessions and the need for insulin climbs up again. From observing the effect of consistent Reiki, she concludes that it enables the body to work more efficiently. She has also noted that the people she works with need to eat after a Reiki session, or they feel dizzy and start to perspire. Her findings have influenced the way I deal with diabetic pets, like Snowball.

I have noticed that pets who receive Reiki regularly from their people, on the order of an hour of *hands on* or *distance* daily, do better than my diabetic clients who receive Reiki from me once a week or less. This shows the value of being steadfast like Tortoise, for as long as the pet's person is faithful to giving decent, daily doses of Reiki, there is the *possibility* that insulin requirements will decrease.

Snowball's blood sugar levels were carefully monitored. In time, she was able to manage well, even when given unrestricted access to a food bowl; so she could eat when her sugar levels began to drop.

I want to emphasize that you should never alter insulin requirements or the diabetic cat's dietary regime without veterinary permission and supervision. Otherwise, you could do great harm to - even kill - your pet. But in those instances where the veterinarian is open-minded and kept involved with the pet through regular clinic visits, and the caregiver is faithful in sharing Reiki, I have seen good things happen. Needless to say, only the most conscientious and dedicated caregivers are able to participate in this way. Not everyone has a schedule that makes this possible. Not everyone is willing to be like Tortoise. And if the pet's person becomes lax about Reiki, the requirements for insulin will rise again. I would rather a pet's person rely solely on drugs and diet to manage this disease, than have the pet's sugar levels seesaw constantly with a varied Reiki regime.

Now, I will only work with diabetic pets if their people have demonstrated mastery of the lesson of perseverance by consistently providing daily Reiki. I prefer that the pet be given a snack after a

85

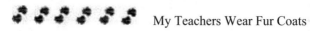

Reiki session to ward off a possible reaction to changing sugar levels. I also insist that a responsible adult stays with the pet for a few hours after such a session, to ensure that she is fine. Thanks to my friend's work with diabetic humans, I'm able to help pets more successfully manage their diabetes as well.

Many pets with chronic illnesses rely more on their people than on me to give them the extended Reiki sessions that they need. Such was the case with Simon, a 16 year old cat who looked like a Holstein cow, with a black mask around his eyes against patches of black and white. His markings were so unusual that he could have won prizes for best pet cat in any cat show. He was troubled by hyperthyroidism, excess secretion of the hormone, thyroxine, which results in an increased metabolic rate. The heart pumps faster, the breathing rate speeds up, as does the functioning of every organ in the body. Left untreated, the animal eats voraciously yet starves to death.

There are three ways to treat such a condition: medication, surgical removal of the thyroid gland itself, or a dose of radioactive iodine. He was initially given medication; it started to make him vomit and was not managing his condition effectively. His status was measured through a blood test of the thyroxine (T4) level. The normal range for a cat ends at 40 nmol/L. His level was over 160 nmol/L and rising. An alternative had to be sought quickly or he would die. He was put on the waiting list at the nearest hospital for radioactive iodine treatment.

In the meantime, he had two, 30-minute *hands on* sessions from his person daily. This might not seem like much compared to the hours of Reiki I mentioned with Friend; but it was all she could manage and she had the commitment of Tortoise. In such situations, consistency is better than sporadic attention.

Each time she shared Reiki with him, she monitored his heart rate with a pediatric stethoscope. She told me that the session had a very specific rhythm. The first 10 minutes felt as if it was taking forever; repeated glances at the clock showed minutes had gone by instead of the hour she felt had passed, as if enormous amounts of Reiki were needed to melt his body's resistance. Yet there was no feeling of vast energy surges coursing through her body, just the perception of time dragging on. About 10 minutes into each session,

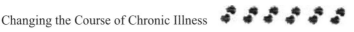

his heart and respiration rates would drop to normal, giving his body a rest. Then his person felt the session fly by and the next twenty minutes felt like three.

When the time came for treatment, Simon was thoroughly examined, with more blood and urine tests, a thoracic x-ray, a cardiac ultrasound, and an electrocardiogram. Test results showed that he was a suitable candidate for radioactive iodine. Between examinations, his person spent five hours a day giving him *hands on* in the hospital. She sent him *distance* for several hours each night.

After the injection of radioactive iodine, he and three other cats with the same treatment were put in an isolation unit for 10 days. During that time, we sent him *distance* for at least two hours daily. To reduce his stress, the staff played a 45-minute tape recording of his person's voice twice a day. Each time Simon heard the tape, he'd start to knead and purr; and it was so soothing that the staff looked forward to switching it on, to relax from a stressful day. Simon responded to the treatment beautifully, looking better than ever by the time he was ready to go home.

About two months later, he went to his veterinarian for the blood test that would show his new T4 level. If the treatment was successful, the level would be close to the normal range. If it was not low enough, it would mean another dose of radioactive iodine was needed. His re-test showed a level of 184 nmol/L, higher than it had ever been! His person insisted on another test in case there was a mistake, but unfortunately, the results were confirmed.

After further consultation between his veterinarian and the veterinary specialist, Simon was x-rayed, for there are times when the treatment fails because of cancer. The x-ray showed a series of grape-like clusters (thought to be tumors) throughout his lungs. His T4 level was rising. There was nothing that could be done.

Simon began to deteriorate; but his person persevered and even increased his Reiki to several hours a day. Regardless of the odds, she was determined to be like Tortoise. He became listless, no longer able to play a game of floor hockey with a tin foil ball. He slept a lot, became less tolerant of touch, and refused to eat. His veterinarian recommended that he be indulged in whatever ways would make him comfortable.

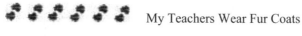

His person cooked him chicken, the only food he seemed able to tolerate. He enjoyed it so much that she started to call him Mr. Chicken. The broth was clarified and reduced into gelatin as a treat. Since his appetite was small, it soon became a treat for all the cats in the neighborhood.

His people's only wish was that he enjoy the summer months, for he liked to lie on the deck baking in the sunlight. His energy levels continued to drop. The amount of Reiki he received was increased again, and he developed a strong preference for it. Anyone who tried to touch him without sharing Reiki was given a swat with his paw.

Then in mid-summer, Simon started to gain weight. He went outside to supervise the vegetable garden. His coat was thick and lush, and his eyes were clear. He seemed more tolerant of touch. By late summer, he was clearly a happy cat enjoying life. So his blood levels were tested yet again, along with another x-ray.

The x-ray was absolutely clear with no sign of those grape-like clusters anywhere. The blood results came a day later; his T4 level had dropped to 54 nmol/L. Later that fall, Simon was re-tested; his T4 was an almost-normal 47 nmol/L and the x-rays were as clear as ever. I think that it was love combined with Reiki that enabled him to pull off this miracle. His person had persevered with Reiki in spite of the dramatic evidence that he was deteriorating. And each time his condition worsened, all she did was increase Reiki and surround him with love. This was a reminder to me that love and devotion in the face of great odds can perform great feats.

On the grounds that all was well, we reduced his Reiki. And all was well for quite some time. We didn't understand that he was not cured but likely in remission; a state where the disease can no longer be detected but may still be lurking. In other words, we made Hare's mistake.

The next spring his person started to sense that Simon's situation was changing, yet his medical tests were as good as ever. Over the summer, her concern continued to build, but she was reluctant to ask for more tests for fear of being branded hysterical. That fall, Simon started to deteriorate. His lungs were fine but there were growths in his abdomen - likely lymphosarcoma. This kind of cancer is terminal, being very reluctant to leave the body.

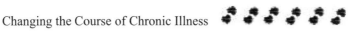

Had I known then what I know now, I would have done two things differently. First, as soon as his medication wasn't working, I would have sent regular *distance* specifically to his thyroid condition, in an effort to help lower his T4 levels. This has worked with some of my clients when Reiki shared in the usual fashion has not yielded results. In these cases, there is a direct relationship between the regular receiving of directed *distance* and the T4 levels. Just as importantly, I make sure that the pet is receiving equal or greater amounts of non-directed Reiki to keep the whole system in harmony. I cannot over-emphasize the importance of this, as I describe further in Chapter Ten. For example, I have worked with Fuzzy, an 18 year old cat who is allergic to hyperthyroid medication and unable to undergo other treatments because of feline leukemia. She receives daily *distance* from me, supplemented by a weekly, in-person visit. We've found that as long as she receives Reiki consistently, her T4 levels remain in the high-normal range. Otherwise, they climb past 100 nmol/L. It is as if by helping to remove some of the stress on the metabolism, the body has enough resources to bring itself back into balance.

Second, I would have strongly recommended that the amount of Reiki be maintained regardless of x-ray and blood results; keeping in mind the potential for remission. It is because of Simon that I truly understood the important of perseverance; but I learned that lesson the hard way, after he had died. Simon taught me that with chronic illnesses, it is better to be like Tortoise, rather than getting off on the adrenaline rush of crisis intervention, like Hare.

Aside from teaching me about his disease, Simon left with me a beautiful memory that captured his struggle against odds that became insurmountable. It was a vision of perseverance, just like Tortoise. Just after he died and I was sending Reiki to his soul, I saw the image of a beautiful flower blooming fully in the sand. The flower, which I took to be Simon, was happy and proud as the sun poured over him like rays of love. One day some sand poured down and bent the flower over, nearly burying it. The flower struggled very hard and straightened himself out. Much later the sand poured down again. The flower kept struggling. Day after day he straightened himself, determined to keep blooming but it was getting more difficult to do so. One night as the brave flower struggled valiantly,

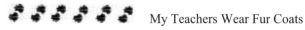

the sand poured non-stop and eventually he lay beneath it. Then, he drifted through a tunnel of light and fully blossomed, radiant in rays of love.

Penny, Friend, Snowball, and Simon have taught me that pets with chronic diseases don't have to face a life of continued discomfort and waning vitality. Careful medical intervention, sensitive monitoring, and Reiki can be powerful adjuncts in supporting their quality of life. With chronic disease, I've learned that consistency and diligence are essential. Especially with Reiki, perseverance regardless of test results can alter the course of the disease, enhancing quality of life and thereby extending its longevity. In fact, many of my clients with kidney disease, diabetes, or hyperthyroidism lead active lives, fully engaged in their world. I see my role and that of their people as being like Tortoise, helping them in the race of life, steadfastly helping them to hold back the progression of chronic illness. I admire their strong spirits blossoming in the sand that surround their lives at this time, and am comforted that they will blossom again when they cast aside bodies that no longer serve them.

Chapter 9

Witnessing the Dance of Death: Lessons in Letting Go

The process of dying is a dance. I call it a dance because it has its own rhythm and set of steps. Sometimes, they are smooth and both the pet and his human partner glide along. At other times, one of the parties finds them difficult to follow, making for a clumsy process, for death, like life, is often imperfect. This dance is all about letting go.

In this chapter, I will talk about the roles I play in the many forms of this dance: how, as with Samara, it can take many turns as the animal dives and rallies; how those like Shiloh are sent to death in despair, while those like Mugsy are blocked from the death they seek. All too rarely, a cat like Cathryn Twinkletoes can show us how everything works out so that both pet and person are at peace. But first, I'll start with Midnight, whose passing embodied the ideal, as her people gently let her go.

Midnight, a dog on the losing end of a battle with cancer, was dying. Her people wanted her to die at home where she could be surrounded by love, and called me for help in her final hours. It was our first and only meeting.

Midnight lay very still. Her breathing was labored. I told her who I was and how I wanted to help her through the transition from her physical form, using Reiki. She accepted and as the sharing of Reiki began her breathing eased. Over the next four hours, she would periodically shift a little to let me know where she wanted my hands placed.

Then she raised her head. Her eyes were filled with love as she gazed at her people. She looked at me; I understood her thanks and request for privacy. I said my farewells and left. Twenty minutes later, I received a phone call letting me know that Midnight had died. She had gone, guided by the gentle love of her people.

Many of us hope that when the time comes, our own pets will leave their form like Midnight did, with peace and dignity. We hope that we will have the strength and maturity of Midnight's people, to surrender our pets to formlessness and memory. If only we knew the exact right time for death, we think we could do it properly.

It is easier to sense that the time for death is drawing near, than to decide when the time for intervention in that process presents itself. Most of us would like death to make its claim without the need of euthanasia, for it is a double-edged gift. It can be an act of kindness, ending the suffering of a beloved pet, but it doesn't make it any easier to let go. Upon reflection, some people believe they used it too soon and should have waited, while others regret that they did not exercise the option sooner. We are each left to our own resources to make that decision. Sometimes we receive the grace to act wisely, as happened with Samara.

Samara is a 20 year old dog who is savoring the process of slowly letting go. With long black hair, white gloves and chest, she is shaped like a bear cub. Yet her bodily housing is deceptive, for underneath it lies a strong determination and love of food that have served her well as she ages.

When she started to slow down a few months ago, she went for a veterinary examination that showed a rapidly growing tumor. Despite her age, her people agreed to surgery knowing that the alternative would be a quick death. To assist her surgical journey, both her person and I used *distance* during the operation and *hands on* after that. Samara came through with flying colors. She continues to receive regular Reiki sessions from her person, supplemented by the occasional one from myself.

One day I arrived for a visit and found a lethargic Samara, unable to eat or walk. Her people wanted to check whether or not these changes signaled her interest in leaving the world, or just a need for extra care. So they began the process of force feeding by putting a syringe of watered-down food (without the needle) in her mouth. To their relief, Samara was willing to swallow the food and water that was offered. To them, it meant she was still interested in living.

We increased her Reiki to daily sessions from both her person and myself, and Samara began to recover. She started to become interested in her surroundings again, looking around and watching where her people were going. Then her appetite returned. Even though she was unable to feed herself, she would direct the syringe with her mouth until it was in the best place for her, wagging her tail as she did so. She began to eat small pieces of dog treats. With increased nourishment, her legs became stronger. To help her walk again, her people held her up by a strong harness so that she could take her steps without the danger of falling.

She is now able to eat solid food, drink water, and walk by herself. The brightness in her eyes has returned and she loves to watch the world around her. Obviously, Samara is not interested in leaving the physical plane just yet. She is fortunate to have people who know her so well and believe in supporting her wishes, rather than deciding that she should move on.

My role with Samara is the same as with any ailing pet: to provide Reiki support as requested. This enables me to get to know the pet quite well and makes it easier to help her, when the time comes to leave her life here. As a witness to the dance of death, I have watched the day-to-day toll of caregiving prove too much for some people to handle, as the pet lurches from crisis to wellness and back to crisis again. In such cases, some people are more than ready to let go: in fact, they give up - as happened with Shiloh.

Shiloh was an elderly dog who was dying from advanced kidney disease. Suddenly, he took a turn for the worse and even with increased Reiki, we were not optimistic. He kept going downhill and by the end of the week, his people made an appointment for euthanasia. Over the next few days, I sent intensive amounts of Reiki to him along with daily visits for *hands on*, and he rebounded.

I'd agreed to attend the euthanasia and we set off in the family car with Shiloh and me in the back seat. As we traveled, I was amazed at how bright and energetic he was, giving me the distinct impression that he still wanted to live. I shared this with his people. "Are you sure he is ready to go? He doesn't seem so, to me."

Finally they retorted, "We don't care whether he is ready or not. The appointment is booked and we're seeing it through."

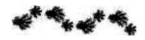

At this point, Shiloh's eyes grew wide. He clung to me and howled. I started to think through my options. It wasn't safe for me to leave a moving vehicle, or to take him with me under the circumstances. Besides, under the law I had no claim to him. All I could do is say, "I'm sorry, Shiloh. There is nothing I can do."

We went into the veterinary clinic. The veterinarian saw the determined looked in the peoples' eyes. Taking into consideration that the dog was elderly and ill, he proceeded to administer the euthanol. I shared Reiki with Shiloh while he died. I was devastated.

It would have been easier on us all if Shiloh had died an unassisted death. In most cases it is a peaceful way to pass on, but it often requires highly attentive care and palliative intervention to keep the pet comfortable as he journeys from his physical form. Without this care and intervention, starvation and dehydration can make it an extremely painful process.

If the person insists on a natural death for his pet, I will encourage him to contact his veterinarian to discuss the implications. And if a cat is involved, I warn his people of the death cry he may give just before he expires. I am not against a natural death, but I find it very difficult to tolerate one that is needlessly painful. And some people are not prepared for the time, financial, and emotional resources needed to provide proper passage.

Many people, like Shiloh's, choose euthanasia instead. Sometimes, the person is so distraught that it is up to me to be the only witness at the euthanasia, though most times my job is to share Reiki while the pet and his person part.

Most euthanasias are a two-step process. First, the pet is taken away to be sedated and have a catheter put in his vein. Especially in older or ailing pets, it can be difficult to find a vein in which to insert the needle, so the process takes place away from the pet's person to lessen the person's distress. During this time, I send *distance*. The pet returns sedated, in the arms of veterinary staff. At this point, I switch to *hands on*. I also start *distance* to the pet's soul. People are usually allowed to spend as much time with their pet as they wish, before euthanol is inserted into the catheter. Based on what euthanized pets have told an animal communicator I know, they feel

an ice cold sensation flooding their veins and stopping their hearts, followed by feelings of peace.

Most times, people are able to spend as long as they wish with their dead pet. They need to take care in holding her at this time, for the body relaxes and fluids leak out. But those who are prepared for this, often want to hold and rock their pet good-bye. She changes dramatically as the soul leaves the body, often to the point of being less recognizable. I continue to send Reiki to her soul.

In Shiloh's case I did not trust my own emotional state, so I phoned a friend to ask her to send Reiki to his soul. She knew nothing of the circumstances around his death. Shortly after, she called me back and asked what had happened, for all she could pick up was despair, grief, abandonment, and betrayal. I explained the situation.

I was angry that Shiloh had been violated and I'd been powerless to stop it. But there were other pets in that household who were frail and needed attention. I didn't think I could afford the luxury of retaliation that would keep me from helping those pets. So I went for a long walk the next day, sending *distance* to his soul. Then I heard a voice with a biblical text about forgiveness, stating that is was up to me to forgive his people because they did not know what they had done. Taking this to mean that Shiloh wanted me to forgive them, I set about that task.

I sent Reiki to myself daily, to the issues around what had happened. Very gradually, I started to experience sadness for his people; for their need to sacrifice such a wonderful dog because they couldn't withstand the demands of his situation. Then came acceptance of what had happened and an understanding of why they had done it: emotional exhaustion from the ups and downs of caring for Shiloh during his cycles of deterioration and rebound, as well as unresolved grief from past deaths. It didn't excuse their actions; it explained them. I released my anger, despair, and judgment, slowly over the course of several months. And while I still believe they made a terrible mistake, the associated venom has gone from my heart. Going through this process of forgiving helped me understand the difference between letting go and giving up.

While some people make the break at a time I sense is too soon, others can't bear to let go. Mugsy's person was one of them. Mugsy was an elderly dog in excruciating pain from crippling, advanced arthritis. He required strong medications and massive amounts of Reiki to keep his pain in check. As the weeks progressed, he became less interested in living: his appetite waned and he spent most of his time sleeping.

When I am working with a pet, like Mugsy, who I already know, I sometimes become aware of the middle of my forehead, the third eye on energetic body maps. When this happens, I know the pet is at a crossroads, deciding whether to live or die. If the sensation becomes more intense, I know that death is favored and if it wanes, it is life. It is my way of monitoring how the interventions taken on the pet's behalf, be they Reiki, medications, or surgery, are affecting the outcome of the pet's decision. I believe that a decision about euthanasia needs to rest with the pet and the pet's person; but sometimes I sense that the two parties are not in agreement. In this case, my forehead and Mugsy were telling me it was time to go. His person had other ideas.

She was having difficulty coping with the loneliness of an empty household now that her husband had followed their adult children out the door. She depended on Mugsy as her only source of support. And because she was so needy herself, she could neither give him the care he needed nor find the courage to let him go. When he refused to snuggle beside her because of his pain, she would forget to feed him or give him his medications. She was never consciously deliberate about this; somehow it just happened. And when this became obvious, I hit the roof.

With the assistance of the dog's veterinarian, we managed to convince his person to make an appointment for euthanasia. And I had a talk with Mugsy. "Mugsy," I said, "it's time for you to start doing what you need to do for yourself. You have taken care of your person for many years. It's time she took care of you." That night and over the next day, Mugsy became increasingly ill. It was obvious even to his person that euthanasia would be an act of kindness.

I accompanied them to the veterinary clinic, sharing Reiki with him, watching his person struggle between doing right by Mugsy and holding on to him even longer. Mugsy was so dehydrated that his veins could not be used for the lethal injection. Instead, euthanol was delivered into his abdominal cavity where it took a while to take effect. During that time his person kept begging Mugsy, "Please don't leave me. Please don't die." And as she said this, I'd feel the push and pull between body and soul: the soul ready to exit his body then suddenly called back to it. So powerful was her hold on him, that he could not leave.

Often when the soul is preparing to leave the body, I have a vision of a seated, robed male figure with bare feet waiting to receive it, surrounded by animals. I know at a deep level that this is Christ. (Perhaps, if my religious background was other than Christian I would see another holy figure instead.) But even though His hand was reaching out to Mugsy, the dog was having difficulty arriving in His lap. I could sense his frustration because my body started to rock, something I've learned is a signal that the pet is at the point of exploding emotionally. I had the horrible feeling that if he continued to be thwarted, his soul would be trapped in limbo. So I sent Reiki to his soul and asked that it do whatever was best for Mugsy.

Then I saw Mugsy in Christ's lap, surrounded by light and my attention shifted back to the room. His body went limp and I was relieved that he was pain-free at last.

People often ask me if I can sense the soul of a being or keep in contact after death. My monitor is that feeling in the middle of my forehead. With pets to whom I am closely bonded, this intensity remains after death for a varying period of time, from several weeks to several months. I send *distance* to the pet's soul every day, until what started as a painful sensation in my forehead slowly ebbs away. When I can no longer feel it, I know that my connection to that soul has been released; and while I am glad to be rid of the pain, I'm also sad at this final loss.

By now you may wonder, has there ever been a death where everything went well? I've been privileged to witness a few of those amongst the many animals I've worked with, including that of Cathryn Twinkletoes, a stunning, cameo-colored cat with eyes the

color of green grapes, who was my feline client and teacher for seven years. She had such regal bearing that I gave her the name, Lady Cathryn, The Lioness. Like royalty at its best, she was discerning about who received her affection. Never a sucker for an open hand or a 'here kitty kitty,' Cathryn viewed you from afar and determined if and when she would deign to brush past your leg in a brief greeting. After I'd won her trust by being circumspect and respectful, she greeted me with resonant purrs especially in response to my stroking her head. Even then, let my hand stray too far down her body when she wasn't in the mood and I'd be corrected with a slap of her paw.

When I stayed with her for several days, Cathryn taught me the virtues of afternoon naps, something she enjoyed, and insisted I join in by leading me to the bedroom and landing on the bed. If I left the room, she left in a huff. I soon learned it was best to lie down.

She also showed me how granting the favor of her companionship could be a sought-for privilege. For example, if I didn't make a sound and kept very still in bed at night, Cathryn would enter the room. I'd hear a mellifluous purr wafting about the room before she'd land on the bed with the gentlest touch. But one move or sound on my part during this process and she'd depart for the evening. Such intermittent reinforcement left me wanting more and so I made sure to keep still for the reward of her companionship.

She set high performance standards and expected them to be met. She ate sparingly in small meals but only if served on clean china and enhanced with fresh toppings, lightly fluffed. She enjoyed the outdoors and expected to be indulged, giving verbal rebuffs if she was taken inside before she was ready. There were times when I failed to meet her expectations and was immediately corrected with her sound of disgust, a quick swat of the paw, or a brief nip. And strange as it may seem, her expectations raised my performance. I'm a sucker for purrs.

Cathryn was plagued by chronic illnesses, at first difficult to discern and diagnose, then morphing into painful bouts of pancreatitis (inflammation of the pancreas) as well as kidney disease. I learned the value of a strong mind in facing challenges, for at times only her determination and strong will kept her alive. When she was

feeling well, she didn't waste time receiving *hands on* but instead paraded about the house and yard while I sent her *distance*. Yet in the midst of a bout of pancreatitis, she'd beckon me over immediately and allow me to touch her most painful areas in expectation that relief would soon follow.

We crisscrossed each others' lives until Cathryn was 19 years old. And I learned a great deal from her. Of all the lessons she taught me, the one I remember best is this: that you can be yourself, warts and all, and still be deeply loved.

Cathryn had a stroke, losing control of half her body. Her person made her as comfortable as possible, following the veterinarian's orders to the letter. We stayed together, sharing Reiki past midnight and I then returned home. There was no improvement. Cathryn was unable to feed herself, drink water without assistance, or use a litter box. The next morning we knew it was Cathryn's last day. We spoke with her through an animal communicator. It became even more obvious that Cathryn was looking forward to being released from a body that was no longer serving her.

I had the privilege of assisting at one of the most peaceful euthanasias ever. Both Cathryn and her person were fully ready and accepted the inevitable, with dignity and peace. Even though more than one try at getting a vein was required, she gave her paw willingly for the needle, without sedation (at her request). Her soul flew out of her body the moment the euthanol touched her vein. We had an instant sense that the very best had happened for Cathryn.

In reflecting on the nature of Cathryn's death, I believe that two things made the difference. The first was that her person had experienced the deaths of three close family members in the previous three years, so she was familiar with loss and the need to let go. She was also prepared to let Cathryn go, having watched her slowly deteriorate over the previous months, accepting the inevitability of her death. She had focused on trying to enjoy each moment with Cathryn, realizing that it could be their last. The second was that she believed Cathryn had as much say in euthanasia as she, her person, did. And when Cathryn showed a readiness to die, both in her behavior and through an animal communicator, her person was willing to accept her decision.

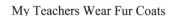

That night, her person and I had a meal in Cathryn's honor. The choice of what to eat was easy, for it was based on one of my strongest memories of Cathryn a week before she died, when she behaved uncharacteristically. That in itself might have warned me that her time was drawing to a close, but I was running late and preoccupied. I decided to pick up a fast food lunch before visiting her. Knowing that Cathryn had no interest in people food, I brought in a cheeseburger and fries. To my surprise, Cathryn went ballistic. She showed so much interest in my lunch that I had to share it, being mindful of her pancreatitis and worrying that such indulgence would set off another attack. So burgers and fries it was on the night she died.

Then we cleared her space at home. This is a request that some people make of me. Others prefer to return home alone, perhaps with a visit from me the next day. Clearing the space, I dispersed any energetic residual related to pain, trauma, or negative energy; it does not mean getting rid of the memory of the pet. In Cathryn's case, I used Reiki symbols and her person used a flower essence preparation called Psychic Spray (the recipe for which is found in Appendix C). The room felt cleaner as a result. She placed a large portrait of Cathryn and some candles on a cupboard in the living room. This became a memorial complete with a beautiful bouquet of flowers sent by her veterinarian. Her person spent the next few weeks making a memorial card and sending it to those who knew Cathryn.

When Cathryn's ashes arrived, her person was not ready to bury them, even though Cathryn had said she wished to be buried in the vegetable garden where she had spent many good summers. A plot was dug and covered with a board, the soil was saved, then winter set in.

On the eve of the Winter Solstice, I attended the committal of her ashes and the celebration of her life. We walked to the graveside in the snow, each carrying a white candle. Words of thanks were spoken and each of us put a memento to rest with her ashes: catnip, her favorite mouse, a piece of her blanket. I put in a piece of cheeseburger and some fries. We left our candles to burn in the soft soil of her grave and sprinkled yellow rose petals as we left.

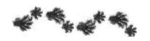

We returned to the warmth of her home with wonderful memories of Cathryn and an eat-with-your-paws tapas feast. Each dish reflected something about Cathryn or one of her companions. We toasted her with champagne and started the feasting with, what else, slices of cheeseburger and handfuls of fries. It was a wonderful tribute to Cathryn Twinkletoes - teacher of pet etiquette, keeper of high standards, and feline friend - who danced so beautifully to her death.

As this chapter shows, the dance of death takes many forms. Each one is a unique opportunity to be tested and held accountable for actions taken. Recently, I have witnessed pairs of deaths that occur a day apart. One day, the dying pet leads the dance according to what I perceive are his wishes; the next day, another pet's wishes are subordinated to those of his person. A wise voice in my head issues a challenge: "This is the way this pet and this person are dancing. It is the way it is and the way it is going to be. Either taint it with your self-righteousness or accept it for what it is." And slowly, I am releasing my ego and surrendering to what is.

In my role as a practitioner, I am sharer of Reiki, witness to the process that connects body and soul, clearer of negativity, mourning support, ritual celebrant, and keeper of memorials. I am recipient of valuable lessons about compassion, forgiveness, loss, and the precious, precarious nature of life. As importantly, the dance of death continues to extend my knowledge of surrender, which runs the gamut from hanging on, to giving up, to letting go.

Part Three:

Lessons From Reiki
With Pets

Chapter 10

Stretching the Canvas of Reiki Practice: Lessons in Questioning

Some of my friends are artists. When they prepare to paint, one of their first tasks is to take wooden stretcher bars and make a frame. That frame sets the limits within which they will paint. But in order to lay color, they need a taut, smooth surface. So they stretch canvas over that frame, holding it to the edge with fasteners. Sometimes they struggle to pull the border of canvas over the edge of the frame. At times, the process of stretching causes the surface to ripple. Then they must remove the fasteners and try stretching it again and again, until the surface is smooth and taut. While stretching canvas is one of the basic tests of committing to art, it is no wonder many artists prefer to use the pre-made version.

The process of stretching canvas is like the process of developing a Reiki practice. Both exist in a state of tension. With canvas, the material is pulled tightly on all sides so that it will form a smooth, strong surface. With Reiki, the foundational principles and attunements are like stretcher bars forming a framework within which Reiki takes place. However, each Reiki student has to use the canvas of instruction or experience to lay the groundwork from which to practise.

Relying on pre-stretched canvas is like accepting your Reiki Master's instruction at face value. And for most of us, that is an excellent choice - most of the time. But in committing to pet-oriented Reiki, I have chosen to stretch my own canvas and, as a result, I create tension as well: between accepted Reiki practice and pet-oriented practice, between what human Reiki Masters have said and what the animals tell me. Under this tension, the process of trying to create a smooth surface from which to work is sometimes tiresome.

105

Sometimes it creates ripples and I have to pull the fasteners that anchor my existing practice out, and start over. Yet even when I redo my canvas, I see myself stretching the fabric of my practice over a solid frame of Reiki.

With any practice, there is a tension between taking something on faith and questioning it. For example, when a student comes to me with a bona fide certificate that states she has a certain level of Reiki, I accept it at face value even if the Master is from a different school. I believe that the person has that Reiki level. Yet when I read that pet-oriented Reiki sessions only take between 10 and 20 minutes because pets are more highly evolved than we are, I feel obliged to test it. Not surprisingly, much of my questioning lies in the realm of practising Reiki with pets, where I have tested a variety of assumptions. They include the following:

> The smaller the being, the shorter the Reiki session.
>
> If you send Reiki to someone under anesthetic s/he will wake up.
>
> Never direct Reiki to a specific disease or body part.
>
> While pets can receive Reiki, they cannot practise it.

In this chapter, I will show how each of these assumptions has caused the canvas of my practice to ripple, beginning with the assumption about size.

The prevailing view of many members of the Reiki community is that small animals only need 10 to 20 minutes of Reiki at the most. Yet in my experience, small beings require as much Reiki as large beings do. Hamsters, birds, kittens, puppies, and cats all benefit from full Reiki sessions just as an adult human does.

The being who most recently supported this finding was Miss Demeanor, a purebred North American Cocker Spaniel puppy born by Cesarean section. She was strong, healthy, and weighed a remarkable 12 ounces; she was a big baby. The following day it became clear that she had problems. She was unable to nurse properly and was defecating from where urine should have streamed. Because she had an incredible will to survive, her person started tube feeding, waiting to see what the future would bring. Reconstructive surgery would be in order if she survived to four weeks of age.

I believe that in situations like this one, it is the being who should decide whether or not to carry on. And since she showed such a strong will to live, I was more than willing to share Reiki with her.

Miss Demeanor needed Reiki and would turn it on full force. She was so small she would curl up into the palm of my hand, cross her front paws over each other, and fall asleep. I would put my other hand over her and Reiki would flow so strongly I would have to ground myself. Indeed, my hands would pulse and grow hot whenever they came close to her.

Sometimes, I would use just one hand while we shared Reiki with her cat companion, Lily Albertina. Despite the difference in relative size, Miss Demeanor would pull the stronger flow through 'her' hand. Lily Albertina did receive some flow too, but definitely not as much as the determined little puppy.

If I had been able to stay with her around the clock, Miss Demeanor would have continued to pull Reiki. Our sessions always ended because I had other commitments, not because she lacked interest. My experience with *distance* was the same: she pulled a strong, powerful flow that never stopped.

Miss Demeanor died when she was 10 days old. Her desire to live continued to the end but her body just couldn't support her spirit, yet she deserved the chance for life that Reiki helped to give her. And whenever someone repeats the myth that small beings should get small amounts of Reiki, Miss Demeanor will support the answer: a resounding "No. Need, not size, determines the length of the Reiki session."

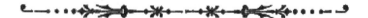

I was warned never to send Reiki to someone under anesthetic because you could wake him up. I took this admonition seriously. Little did I realize that others might not. I found this out when my cat, Beakers, was very ill and required surgery, even though his veterinarian was not confident that he would pull through. I accepted the offer of a friend to send him some Reiki. I gave her the surgery time so she could work around it, sending *distance* before his operation and when it was finished. But she had completely forgotten the admonition about not sending Reiki to beings under anesthetic, and so she proceeded to send it at the exact time he was under the knife.

We wouldn't have been the wiser if it was not for Beaker's veterinarian who took me aside and asked, "Did you do anything while Beakers was being operated on?"

"What do you mean?" I asked.

"You know, that thing that you do."

"Ah, Reiki. No I never sent him any Reiki. Why did you ask?"

"When we put him under anesthetic his vital signs became weak and unstable. This had me worried. Then all of a sudden, all his vital signs improved, stabilized, and remained so for the operation."

Later that day, I told my friend of the conversation. She replied, "You told me when he was being operated on, so I sent it for that time. In fact, I thought you'd send him some, too."

From then on, I've been comfortable sending Reiki to animals under anesthetic, confident that it will support them without interfering in any negative way. In fact, by sharing Reiki in this way, many animals who faced high-risk surgery have been helped. It was a blessing that my friend's memory was so short that she unknowingly tested the assumption about anesthetic, for I would have never tested the admonition for fear of the consequences. I now know that sending Reiki to animals under anesthetic is as helpful as sending to them when they are awake.

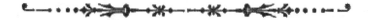

Reiki seems to have a wisdom of its own and directs itself to where it is most needed. That is why I, along with many others, have been taught to send Reiki to wherever it is needed, but not to otherwise direct it. This was a practice to which I adhered until I hit a brick wall with a pet who was in excruciating pain that was not responding to Reiki. His name was Higgins.

Higgins (whom I mentioned in Chapter Three) was a handsome orange cat with long, silky fur and a tail like an ostrich plume. He was the leader of a multi-cat household and would inspire the other

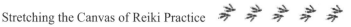

males to feats of mischief, like going into the basement and digging through boxes of Christmas decorations or indulging in games of chase. And whenever two cats in the household disagreed, Higgins was there to settle the argument. The only fly in the ointment was pancreatitis, a debilitating inflammation of the pancreas often triggered by rich or fatty food; yet it can strike without warning and the pain can be excruciating. To make matters worse, Higgins was afflicted at a time when veterinarians thought that only dogs, but not cats, could be afflicted with the disease. Needless to say, no conventional treatment was available. Fortunately, Higgins had access to a veterinary homeopath whose remedies kept him well for over a year.

One day Higgins drank a small amount of milk, setting the scene for another attack. But this one was much worse. His person started him on his remedy, but it didn't work. She called the homeopath, but any suggested remedy failed.

His conventional veterinarian was convinced it was inflammatory bowel disease and recommended he be taken to a veterinary specialist - an eight-hour drive away. But his person was convinced it was pancreatitis and she knew that the treatment for inflammatory bowel disease would make it worse. In desperation, she began working with another veterinarian and thanks to connections in the United States, found out that there was a new test to determine the presence of pancreatitis: the Trypsin-like Immunoreactivity Test or TLI. Higgin's blood was sent to Texas, the only place where the test was done and the diagnosis was confirmed: pancreatitis. He was given intravenous fluid to restore his hydration and provide him with some nourishment. However, there was no cure and the bout would not abate.

His person was beside herself. "I just know he is going to die and there is nothing I can do about it," she would often say. She called me and arranged for mega Reiki sessions. Higgins received about seven hours a day of *distance* targeted specifically to his pancreas, because that was the only thing that seemed to give him any relief. But sending Reiki to him did not have the impact we had hoped. Moreover, he could not tolerate *hands on* because the pressure from even light contact was far too painful. Instead, he liked

109

to sit in the enclosed hollow at the base of a large cat tree to receive *distance* Reiki directed to his pancreas. I reasoned that the hollow would fill with Reiki and keep him comfortable long after I left. The pain lessened and Higgins seemed to have turned a corner.

One of the greatest challenges was to get Higgins to keep his food down. Even when he had an appetite, he would soon vomit his food back up. I tried using *hands on* to help with this and there were no results. *Distance* sent specifically to his pancreas was a great help in relieving his pancreatic pain, but did nothing for nausea. I knew he continued to be nauseated because he would hunch up, keeping his neck extended; and sometimes he would gulp air or pant, as well. One day I decided to send Reiki by *distance* directly to his nausea condition. I felt his nausea and then it abated. About an hour after that *distance,* he was able to eat and keep his food down. This kind of *distance* was a breakthrough for both of us.

I wish I could say that all was well after that. However, he started to become dehydrated and needed extensive subcutaneous hydration. Was it the large volumes of Reiki coupled with his lack of interest in water? (Now, I'm always insistent that a pet has free access to water during and after Reiki.) Or was it the sign of his body trying to achieve balance and going out of whack instead? Regardless of the possible explanations, this seesaw continued and his person was ready to stop the Reiki for fear it was the cause. But then Higgins turned the corner again and all seemed to be well. He was looking better, showing an interest in moderate portions of food, and even beginning to play.

His person took him for a veterinary checkup. There was a lump in his stomach that had never been found in all the numerous checkups he had received over the past three months. So exploratory surgery was scheduled four days later. By this time Higgins was in full swing, enjoying life and playing his favorite game - batting at water flowing down the drain. At last, his person truly felt things were going to go well.

By the time he went for surgery, the tumor had burst, spreading the cancer throughout his body. It had invaded every organ, except one: his pancreas. Higgins was euthanized while under anesthetic. His person was devastated. And I was left wondering if so specifically targeting the Reiki had been such a good idea.

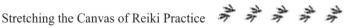

I had believed I was doing my best for Higgins and obviously it worked; it just didn't help save his life in the face of a cancer no one knew he had. Yet it is not unusual for a pet to have conditions of which I have no awareness, that can override any good I am trying to do.

I am reminded of the old adage: Be careful for what you wish, you might get it. We are often quite clear about what we want but, because we are missing many of the facts, we don't really know what we need. This is why the best prayers express requests by asking for what is best for us in the largest scheme of things, tempered with thanks for what we have already been given. In Higgin's case, Reiki went to where it was needed; but it was needed in so many places at once (the cancer, the pancreas, the nausea) that it could not build up enough intensity at any one spot to make an apparent difference. It's as if against such odds, the Reiki spreads itself too thin or bounces from place to place because it is needed everywhere. When I directed it exclusively to his pancreas in an attempt to focus its healing power, it did just that but only that. I've learned that interfering with Reiki in this way is risky and dangerous.

Taking this lesson into account, I still direct Reiki in specific situations where I have found it to yield better results than Reiki sent in the usual fashion: hyperthyroidism, pancreatitis, nausea, and temporomandibular joint dysfunction (TMJ), with two important changes. *First, I never direct Reiki on a regular basis unless the pet is also receiving an equal or greater number of Reiki sessions that are done in the usual fashion, as well. And I ask that Reiki be sent to the core problem of the entire condition, rather than to a specific organ.* In these ways, I try to balance out what the pet's person and I believe to be in the pet's best interests, with where the Reiki wishes to go. Energetically, I am hedging our bets. In other words, I believe that Reiki can be directed to specific ailments or body parts; however, because of the limits of human knowledge about the pet and whole condition, it is wise to ensure an equal or greater number of regular Reiki sessions as well, bowing to the limitations of our knowledge.

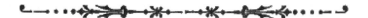

Reiki cannot be learned from a book. You must be initiated by a Reiki Master. While most Masters restrict this initiation to humans, some include pets as well, which means that the pet is then capable of sending Reiki to others.

After hearing about this for several years, my curiosity got the better of me and I decided to see if my cats could be initiated. I wasn't a Master at the time so a friend gave them their Level One (the ability to send Reiki *hands on*, or should we say, *paws on*), after which I contacted an animal communicator to check things out.

My eldest cat, Friend, was thrilled and began calling herself a Reiki Master. Kahlua, my energy-sensitive Siamese-cross was ambivalent. And Christmas Blessing, my youngest and most emotionally vulnerable cat, was distressed by what he called his toes of light. I explained what had happened and although he understood it, he was not happy. Only then did I realize the mistake I had made: not receiving their informed consent before I went ahead. This was truly a case of my curiosity taking precedence, and it was disrespectful and unfair. After all, who am I to decide some being should become a Reiki channel?

Since then, I have been asked by some caregivers to initiate their pets to Reiki and almost always have refused. My main reasons are that I have no behavioral evidence of the pet's interest in learning Reiki and no evidence of consent. Without it, the process is coercive, counter to the spirit of Reiki.

To date, I have no evidence that the cats with whom I live are practising Reiki. I have, however, initiated two littermates, Beauty and Timmy, with their consent, strange though this may sound. Beauty with her short, chocolate-black fur distinguished with a tuft of white on her belly has golden eyes that mirror the intensity of a dedicated Reiki student. Timmy is the charming orange and white tabby I described in Chapter Seven, who suffers from lymphosarcoma, a terminal form of cancer. Since their person received her Level One Reiki, both cats have Reiki every day. Beauty draws Reiki strongly and loves being held to receive *hands on*, while Timmy is largely a *distance* man. About a year later, their

112

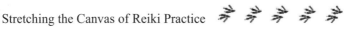

person talked with them through an animal communicator who transmitted Beauty's request to learn what I do, that is, Reiki, so she could help her companion. Her person was taken by surprise. She also checked with Timmy who was not as eager to learn, but was fine with it. Because I knew their caregiver well and sensed her honesty, and knew and respected the particular animal communicator she used, I went ahead and initiated both cats. She was thrilled and he was okay. Now Timmy shares Reiki from time to time, but Beauty has become quite masterful.

When Timmy is having a bad day, Beauty snuggles into him, all four paws in direct contact with his body, Reiki-ing him away. At a recent Reiki circle, a meeting of initiates to share Reiki, I was lying on my stomach on the couch in Beauty's living room ready to receive Reiki to my lungs, the source of my asthma. Beauty lay on my back and I felt two, tiny flows from her front paws and a large one from her abdominal area where she'd tucked her hind feet.

Beauty's caregiver attests to Beauty's use of Reiki for healing her as well. She knows when Beauty is sending *distance* because the cat sits on the back of the sofa with her paws purposefully placed in front of her. Sometimes when Beauty receives *hands on,* she'll send that person *distance* at the same time. My most recent experience came after falling on the ice and hurting my knee. When I saw Beauty later that day, she came over and sniffed up and down my legs until she'd found the exact source of the pain. There she sat down, purred, and began Reiki. I felt a strong flow and the pain receded.

Beauty has continued with Reiki and now has her Level Three. Through an animal communicator she has said she particularly enjoys being able to do Reiki herself. It makes her paws tingle and sparkle. And she feels bigger, as if she is at a higher vibrational level.

Beauty is one of a number of cats known for sensing changes in the energy field of other beings and doing something to normalize them. The probable explanation for this has many strands: the cat's territorial nature, her sensitivity to energy fields, her ability to purr, and in Beauty's case, her knowledge of Reiki.

113

We know that cats place a high value on territory. It is so important to them that they will go without food, sleep, or sex in order to secure it. The core territory (where the cat eats, sleeps, and eliminates) is frequently patrolled and scent-marked to let others know of the cat's presence and just as importantly, give a sense of comfort by being surrounded by her own smell - much the same as we strew our possessions about to make a place feel like home. In domestic situations, people and other pets are part of a cat's territory and get marked too; the cat rubs against them and deposits chemical markers called pheromones.

Changes to the territory can induce anxiety in a cat because a change may mean bad news, for example that the food supply is threatened or that the sleeping area is no longer safe. One such change can be a disruption of the energy field belonging to a being in the territory.

Each living being has its own energy field. When that being is well, the field is smooth. When the being is not well, the field changes. People who work with energetic forms of healing can note changes in temperature, texture, or flow over particularly troubled areas. Some energy workers describe painful areas as feeling hot, sticky, and jagged, almost like static.

Cats can sense energy even at a distance. When I use *distance* with a cat in the same room, say 10 or 20 feet away, the receiver will often come up to my hands, look them over carefully, sniff between them and do the Flehmen response (a sort of sniff/taste since cats can actually taste smells) and then walk away - only to return to the hands several times during the session. There is nothing visible between my hands though I can sense a ball of energy, so I conclude that the cat is sensing the concentration of energy between my hands. It follows that it would be easy for a cat to sense an energetic disturbance and attempt to normalize it, to bring the territory back in line. And purring is one way to do so.

Cats purr between 27 and 44 Hertz (or cycles per second). The purr has recently been discovered to be a self-healing mechanism in cats (though it does have other uses, as well). We know that vibrations of 20 to 50 Hertz help human bones get stronger and grow, as does ultrasound used after acute, and with chronic injury. Even low intensity ultrasound can have a positive effect on tissue.

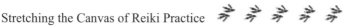

When a cat puts her purring body in contact with yours, she is sharing that healing vibration.

Thus the cat has the ability to sense the energetic disturbance, locate it exactly, and then purr it away. And most of the other cat healers of whom I am aware do so by sniffing the general area until the exact spot is found, then sitting on it, and purring until the pain recedes. But Beauty adds another dimension, her Reiki, which I feel as a distinct flow into my body when she shares it with me. Beauty is a therapist extraordinaire.

I have no idea whether or not Beauty does self-treatments. I have seen her curled up with her paws tucked against her body, but that is such a standard cat position that it is difficult to say. However, she does receive Reiki on a regular basis from her person: one healing attunement a day plus whatever *hands on* she wishes, in addition to hitchhiking on the *distance* her person sends to others. This is important because Beauty has a number of health challenges of her own: mild kidney disease, a thyroid condition that goes out of whack from time to time, inflammatory bowel disease, and a history of nasty bladder infections. I can only hope that her new-found ability to transmit Reiki will enable her to help herself, as well as the other pets and humans with whom she chooses to share it.

Beauty showed me that Reiki works through intent, that by being initiated, the sender's intent is always to send Reiki to heal the receiver. Because I don't know how Beauty might manage to say a mantra and I've never seen her wave her paws to make a symbol, I understand that these are optional tools for focusing intent; they to not replace it. She has taught me that a pet can be a Reiki initiate. And I'm sure that if I asked her about such initiation, she'd tell me to go ahead - but only if I was sure I had the animal's full consent.

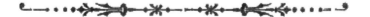

I've had the opportunity to re-stretch the canvas of my Reiki practice with experience. Each time the canvas starts to ripple or the surface is no longer taut, I know it is time to question my assumptions. There are many parts of my canvas that have always remained taut; these I accept at face value. But let the surface slacken and to take the risk of asking yet another question. I feel free to test all the rules and admonitions, letting the animals teach me what works and doesn't work with Reiki, though it isn't always a comfortable process. And I'm confident that at least for me, the following applies:

Share Reiki based on need, not size, of the recipient.

It is safe to share Reiki with pets under anesthetic.

It is more efficient to direct Reiki to a specific disease or bodily condition under certain circumstances, as long as you provide an equal or greater number of general Reiki sessions to ensure that the full being is not neglected.

Initiate pets to Reiki only if certain of their consent; that likely means that such Reiki students will be few and far between.

Chapter 11

Following A Reiki Path: Lessons in Becoming

Having a Reiki practice is different from living a Reiki life. On the one hand, a practice refers to the sharing of Reiki usually in exchange for remuneration. It becomes a form of livelihood, perhaps a vocation. On the other hand, living a Reiki life requires that you live in a way that contributes to harmony and balance, according to certain principles or precepts. There are five principles that have been variously translated and provide the foundation for living a Reiki way of life. They can be summarized as follows:

Present-centeredness. Don't concern yourself with the future or worry about the past. Live in the present, a day at a time.

Peace. Curb your anger and set your hard feelings aside, so that you live in calm and inner peace, day by day.

Honest Livelihood. However you earn your living, do so with integrity, being fair and open in your dealings.

Honor. Respect those who have guided and continue to guide you; recognize the value of their teachings.

Kindness. Treat everything that lives with good will and generosity.

These precepts provide a framework for living a meaningful life. My students receive a printed sheet of these principles over a background image of my cat, Kahlua, the mascot of my business. Having a pet on such a page gently reminds them of their

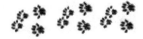

commitment to the animal world. The precepts are deceptively simple and truly sophisticated. Easy to grasp on the surface, they provide a lifetime of guidance and can take more than a lifetime to master. To commit to living a Reiki life means trying to embody Reiki in every thought, feeling, and action, thereby manifesting its principles through just being.

In this chapter, I'll share what Ginger has taught me about worry, through present-centeredness; how Beakers and Sara have tried to teach me about peace when I'm feeling angry; how my animal companions have forced my honesty - holding me accountable for the way I practise my livelihood; how I have learned to honor one of my teachers, Little Lady, in the way I conduct my business; and how pets like Seraphim give me the opportunity to show kindness.

Present-centeredness.
Don't concern yourself with the future
or worry about the past.
Live in the present, a day at a time.

Ginger was a handsome cat with a shorthaired, orange-and-white coat who shared his life with several companions: a feisty, feline female; assorted Cocker Spaniels; a Greyhound; and a human being. He had all the advantages of living on an acreage - a warm place to sleep, plenty of food, and the chance to roam outside during the day in relative safety.

We became very well acquainted as we worked together to support his kidneys, already quite diseased, and his mouth, which had a nasty cancer. As a result, he had high Reiki requirements: *hands on* six days a week, and *distance* three to four times daily. In good weather, I would begin our sessions with a mug of coffee because caffeine keeps my asthmatic bronchial tubes relaxed so I wouldn't upset him with coughing. We'd head outside where I would sit and chat with him - me drinking my coffee and him soaking in the sun's rays and roaming about. I stayed overnight when his person was away and my cats would stay in another part of the house. He seemed to know that I wouldn't let my cats out until

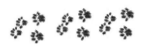

he had had his fill of the outdoors and was ready to go inside. And as if he knew they were waiting, he would stretch his outdoor visits even longer when they stayed over, the little stinker. You should have heard the grumbling from my own tribe!

I learned that Ginger's Reiki requirements could not be scrimped on or he would deteriorate. At times, they needed to be increased to meet the seriousness of his health issues. This became particularly pronounced as the cancer spread in his mouth making eating more difficult, and to his eye, putting more pressure in his head.

In spite of all the challenges, Ginger enjoyed life. He continued to be interested in the world around him. He had a healthy appetite. He taunted his cat companion. He supervised dog grooming. And he was particularly proud when he caught mice.

We had several opportunities to talk through an animal communicator. He never admitted to being sick and refused to discuss his health. In his view, it was a closed subject. He was very aware of the limited time he had left in his physical form and he wanted to make the most of it.

That didn't prevent me from thinking about his future and about my future without him. Whenever my mind wandered in this way, I would feel sad. Lost in such thoughts, I'd become aware of a very annoyed-looking Ginger gazing intently at me. It was as though he was saying, "Susan, I'm *still* here. Let's enjoy the here-and-now and let the future take care of itself." Then I would smile at him and tell him I was sorry. He'd accept my apology with purrs, rubbing up against me, signaling me to follow him so he could show me something of interest. And now, I am without my acreage tour guide and I miss him.

In reflecting on our time together, I am grateful that he allowed me to have a deeper understanding of the Reiki precept on present-centeredness. He had a strong desire to live in the present and an equally strong desire to keep me present-focused. His philosophy of living enabled him to drink in all the experiences that presented themselves and trust that the future would take care of itself. In following his advice, I was able to share his delight in life and enjoy some of the experiences he treasured, leaving me with more

119

wonderful memories than I would have had if I'd continued to indulge my future-focus.

As the end of his time with us drew near, Ginger looked forward to being released from his physical form. He was in a very good mood the day he died, enjoying every moment, trusting in the future that awaited him.

He taught me the value of staying in the present and enjoying the abundance that life has to offer. He taught me the value of not wasting time focusing on things over which I have no control. And so I will always think of Ginger when I review the Reiki precept of present-centeredness.

Peace.
Curb your anger and set your hard feelings aside,
so that you live in calm and inner peace, day by day.

This second precept, about peace, is the most difficult one for me. I've had firsthand experience with deep anger and what I learned was this: the more I kept my anger inside myself, the more I took it out on myself; and the more I allowed it to rise to the surface, the more violent I became. Regardless of the popular opinion that letting it hang out is a good thing, doing just that was my recipe for disaster. So I've done my best to avoid anger at all costs, it being a very dangerous enemy for me.

For a long time, I've admired beings who can handle anger by letting it out in a prompt, clean fashion, who just get it over with. The prime example of this was my cat, Beakers, a distinguished and diminutive chocolate-point Siamese who had the bearing and emotional volatility of an Italian count. He lived in the same house whose basement I rented. Four times he was adopted by people who moved out and didn't take him along, leaving him a twofold legacy before his first birthday: a fondness for beer and a fear of being abandoned.

My heart went out to this tiny critter, so I invited him to join my family. Once that was clear, Beakers became the major domo of my household even to the point of selecting our next family member, a small mackerel tabby kitten I named Beaker's Friend. We became

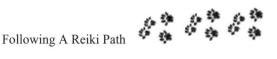

close, yet when it was time for me to move, Beakers became distressed. He cried, dragging his belly along the floor and urinating as he went. Obviously, he figured I would be another one in a long line of fickle guardians. It took several moves before Beakers fully realized that he and I were a package deal and wherever I was going, he'd be going too.

He loved wandering about the neighborhood and visiting with other cats until his outdoor adventures were curbed by the development of glaucoma. Not only was it misdiagnosed, but the medications to deal with it were ineffective. Though Beakers lost both eyes, he gained the ability to see into your soul. His sockets were closed over in a field of dark brown fur giving him a peaceful, penetrating gaze resembling the wise Yoda of Star Wars fame.

I was just starting my Reiki practice. To supplement my income, I did petsitting, some of which involved overnight stays. I would pack my bag but leave my cats in the apartment. I'd visit them once or twice a day or make arrangements for other friends to provide them with company.

Beakers felt strongly about my absences and even more so when he'd lost his eyes. Perhaps it was because of his Siamese background - since it is the cat breed most prone to separation anxiety. Perhaps it was his past history. It may very well have been his way of warning me that I'd better get out of the petsitting business and on to Reiki full-time. In any event, he developed a ritual that marked my re-entry into the household.

When I'd return for good, the cats would know it by the presence of my overnight bag steeped in new smells. Beakers would address me with a series of invectives in Siamese - yelling up one side of me and down the other. Then he would go to the living room rug and squat. When he arose there would be one, and only one, turd in the middle of the carpet. Off he'd walk, satisfied that he'd made his point. And then we were friends again.

There are many theories about anger. Some say it is best to get it out. Beakers showed me that if anger cannot be contained, then release it and be free. His anger was short-lived. He didn't let it fester. He said what he felt, loudly and clearly. I admired his honest

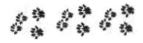

expression of emotion because it meant that he could leave his anger behind (quite literally) and get back to loving me. Yet, in spite of the clarity of his example, I am not the type who can release my anger so easily.

Another way of dealing with anger is through goodwill, that is, by showing compassion, mercy, and love. And my best teacher for that has been Sara. She showed me the power of love in the face of emotional difficulties; anger is certainly emotionally difficult for me.

Sara was a sad, withdrawn, 18 year old cat with advanced kidney disease. While I was hired to provide support to her ailing body, I was haunted by her sadness. I sent her all the Reiki she wanted but it didn't make the difference for which I hoped. She responded best when, during *distance,* I drew the mental/emotional symbol I learned from Level Two Reiki over her. One day as I was sending Reiki to Sara, I was inspired to add the message: sending hearts full of love and Reiki. I'm a kinesthetic and auditory person, so I just felt the hearts and spoke the message silently, though I have a vague sense that these hearts come in a variety of colors.

After that, Sara started to blossom, becoming more engaged in life and interested in play. Now, whenever I meet pets who are troubled - sad, timid, insecure, lonely, unwanted, or nearing the end of their lives - I think of Sara and send them hearts of love.

I had never thought of applying hearts of love to the feeling of anger, until I found myself in a situation of deep rage, afraid to unleash it because it felt it could never be contained and afraid to suppress it lest it eat me up inside. I know that when anger affects me in this way, it siphons the joy out of my heart, leaving it an emotional desert. In the course of several self-treatments, I came to understand that sending hearts of love can water my arid heart.

Love has many dimensions. It includes forgiveness, exudes kindness, and is generous in its mercy. Most of all, it is restorative. Slowly, I am learning that by restoring my inner peace through self-treatments dosed liberally with hearts of love, I can greet those situations that vex me with restraint, forbearance, and goodwill. With time, I might be able to show them some affection, grounded in a sea of calm.

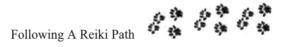

Honest Livelihood.
However you earn your living, do so with integrity,
being fair and open in your dealings.

The precept on livelihood has made my vocation of sharing Reiki with pets a challenging one, for there have been times when the teachings of my human guides have differed from those of my animal teachers. The animals have prevailed.

Choosing to work with Reiki and pets was a long process. Even though pets have always been my closest friends, I did not plan on a future working with animals.

During young adulthood, I began to experience flashbacks, glimpses of repressed traumatic memories. I burned my arms with lit matches. After six years of intensive therapy, the memories were cleared. Yet my pent up anger was escalating along with my harm to my arms. I saw a physiotherapist and a massage therapist to help rectify this self-inflicted damage, but their methods terrified me. I was told to consider something less invasive. "What about Reiki?" someone suggested.

I started with one-hour Reiki sessions five days a week. Each was painful, traumatic, and exhausting. Only my faith that this would help me, kept me going. For the first six weeks, I would allow only my arms to be touched, and it was six months before I had the kind of Reiki session that most people report from the first: a blissful, relaxing experience. A few months later, I let my arms heal completely.

While my pets comforted me throughout my healing journey, the issue of finding a livelihood came up repeatedly. The first sense of my true vocation came after I received my Level One Reiki (Usui Shiki Ryoho, 1994) which enabled me to treat myself. And to this day, self-treatment is my foundation. With Level One, my hands and arms were no longer the repository of past trauma; being healed, they became a vehicle for healing.

In retrospect, it was only natural for me to focus this gift on the strongest allies in my healing journey: my pets. Yet at first I didn't make the connection between pets coming up to me and putting their

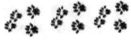 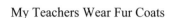

bodies under my hands, with the possibility of earning a living in this way. Although they were telling me that I'd found my vocation, it took a vivid dream in which I was given the phrase, "Reiki for pets in the comfort of their home" and two symbols side-by-side - an animal's paw and a human palm, for me to get the message. These words and symbols became the basis of my business card and because they were so powerful and precious to me, I had them trademarked.

Two months later, Muffy, my brother's Terrier-cross, and Tabby, my mother's Cockapoo, confirmed my true vocation when they were seriously injured by another dog. By the time I found out about their condition, they were at the veterinary clinic and it was closed. I had to wait until the next day to share Reiki because I only had Level One and thus could not do *distance*. Tabby died that night. Then and there I decided that I needed Level Two, which would enable me to share Reiki without physical contact.

Meanwhile, Muffy needed 61 stitches. The veterinarian said that if she survived, reconstructive surgery would be required. With veterinary permission, I gave her Reiki during her hospitalization. She healed rapidly without the need for further surgery. This reinforced a feeling deep within me that I could share Reiki with pets as a form of what Buddhists call right livelihood.

I started seeing other animals on a no-charge basis. Through veterinary recommendation, I got my first paying client: Tess, a Golden Retriever with a hemorrhage in her back right leg, who was in such pain that neither she nor her people were getting much sleep. During the weeks before an accurate diagnosis could be made, she managed her pain through Reiki. Soon, both she and her people were sleeping through the night. Then I gave her several Reiki sessions to prepare her for surgery and for her recovery from leg amputation. She recovered much more quickly than expected because Reiki enhanced her body's ability to heal itself. It also made a difference to her people because it was obvious that she enjoyed receiving it.

That's how I knew I'd found my calling. It took me four more years before I was able to give up the various part-time jobs I used to support myself, to devote all of my working life to Reiki. Throughout that time, I kept getting visual images both of working

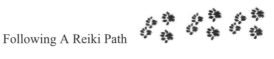

with pets and also of initiating people to Reiki in their homes. So I became a Master's apprentice.

During my apprenticeship, a sense of urgency started to build inside me. Victoria (the Cocker Spaniel described in Chapter Seven) was starting to need six hours of Reiki a day to control the bleeding from her rectal tumor. I was having difficulty accommodating this need into my schedule. Then a friend, who had just received Mastery from another Reiki school, told me about the healing attunement. Unlike the attunements received by a student from a Master in order to be initiated to the different levels of Reiki, this one is solely for the purpose of intensifying healing. According to her, such an attunement would significantly reduce the amount of Reiki needed.

I asked her to do a healing attunement with Victoria. It was sufficient to stop her bleeding for a day. Intrigued, I asked her to work with another of my clients. Again, I was impressed by the speed at which change occurred. I wasn't completely comfortable with the healing attunement process but the results it enabled were so striking that I wanted to use it. I felt strongly that this was a technique I needed to have, now. But it was not taught by the school in which I was enrolled. (In time, my animal teachers showed me how to change the way I do healing attunements and the circumstances under which I do them.) Caught between a rock and a hard place, I made a decision to further my work on pet-oriented Reiki at the expense of rupturing my relationship with my highly-esteemed Master.

Because I continued to get visions of initiating people with pets to Reiki, I enrolled with another Master who agreed to teach me, using only the four symbols originally discovered by Dr. Usui and nothing more. After being initiated as a Master/Teacher (Traditional Japanese Reiki, 2000), I became independent of any Reiki school. Now I am able to fulfill my original vision: being able to share Reiki with pets and teach a pet's person Reiki, in his own home.

Becoming an independent Master/Teacher is the price I pay for forging my own Reiki path. This means that I have no formal relationship with a person to whom I can turn for guidance. Yet every session I do is a learning opportunity. And sometimes these

125

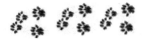

opportunities come in bunches. For example, when I first started my practice, I shared Reiki with a series of animals all of whom died. While it was a privilege to witness their journey, it was also discouraging. I felt like I was bringing them the hands of death. The voice inside me asked, "Are you willing to commit to a Reiki practice, even if the results are not as you might wish?" When I made that commitment, I encountered another series of pet clients presenting another lesson.

The next lesson was taught by pet lovers, rather than the pets themselves. With the next group of clients, all of their people were eager to arrange Reiki sessions. All of their people acknowledged the positive changes that these sessions had made for their pets. All of them were financially able to continue. And all of them cancelled Reiki after four or five sessions. The common obstacle was priorities: none of the people could arrange their schedules to accommodate their pets. Again, I was issued a challenge since the reason for stopping the sessions made no sense to me and did not fit my value system. Was I willing to stick with a Reiki practice, even if I had no control over whether or not sessions continued? Upon reflection, I agreed to carry on. In this way, I have plenty of opportunities to learn.

I also depend on Sara and Beakers, even though they no longer have physical form. They have taken on the responsibility for my continued education and personal development, as well as my protection.

When I am exhausted and driving late at night, Beakers appears in the corner of my eye to warn me, just before I drift over an embankment. He also gives me direction in particular situations.

He can be unrelenting in his efforts to guide me. For example, I received a call from a former client who lives with a dog and a cat. While both animals are loved and cared for, the dog is the center of her life. That day, her dog started limping for no apparent reason, so she requested a Reiki session. When I arrived a few hours later, the dog stopped limping - before the session had begun.

In the course of my visit, I noticed that his cat companion was seriously ill. Their person acknowledged that while she knew the cat

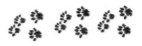

was ill, no veterinary clinic would help her because she didn't have any money. I sympathized with her and left.

I was only two blocks away from their home, when I heard a nagging Siamese voice in my head. It was Beakers telling me I could not walk away. And anyone who has heard a Siamese cat insistent on getting his way, will know that it is difficult to ignore. To stop his nagging, I arranged for the cat to be temporarily transferred into my care, so I could make all medical decisions and pay for them using the services of my own veterinarian. It took a while to convince the person to trust me, for she feared that I wouldn't return her cat, even if she recovered. But Beakers kept nagging me to persist. So I told her that her dog, the apple of her eye, was worried about the cat - so worried that he faked his limp just so she would call me. And when he knew I would arrive, his mission was completed and he stopped limping. I went on to say that Beakers was taking over and making sure the dog's wishes were carried out. Then I said, "Your dog cares about what happens to his cat companion. He wants help for her. Are you going to say 'no' to him?" She released the cat into my custody.

The cat recovered and returned to her home. But Beakers was not content with my just taking action. He wanted me to reflect on the situation and understand it more deeply. Beakers was telling me that there are cases where I have a spiritual responsibility, even though I may not be the pet's legal guardian. It was a sobering lesson.

Working with Reiki and pets is my way of giving back the gift of healing to those who stood by me when I most needed it. My Reiki practice and its distinctive style owe their existence to a consortium of animals who have chosen to show me the pet-oriented Reiki way, either by presenting themselves for sessions or by taking on the senior roles of guide and protector, much the same as any Reiki Master would do.

As a result, I accept as students anyone interested in learning about pet-oriented Reiki. Almost always, I refer those who want Reiki for themselves or other humans, to other Masters. When I teach, animals are always present; my own pets work with my students from time to time. Based on what animals have taught me, I

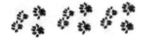

do four attunements for a Level One initiation, believing that they offer the necessary protection to keep both the transmitter and receiver of Reiki safe from harm. Almost without exception, I teach the healing attunement (which I term, Level Three) only to those people whose pets are ill enough to require it. Until I meet someone willing to invest in the hours of apprenticeship with animals that I believe are necessary, I will not initiate anyone as a Master/Teacher.

Animals have encouraged me to travel a Reiki path and I have chosen to heed them. The way I teach and the lessons I learn are based on my experiences with pet-oriented Reiki; they are not all there is to know. In traveling this path, I believe I am engaging in honest livelihood: true to animals, true to Dr. Usui's teachings, and true to myself. My practice is my truth.

Honor.
Respect those who have guided and continue to guide you;
recognize the value of their teachings.

The fourth Reiki principle is about honor, respecting my guides. It will come as no surprise that most of my guides have been pets. In deference to their gifts to me, the buffet in my dining area houses their mementos: figurines, small photos, clippings of their fur, and other material items that symbolize our relationship. When I walk past this area, I remember the special times we shared. I have photos of most of the pets with whom I have worked, so I can enjoy being surrounded by good friends and take comfort in the guidance they have given me. And I honor every pet I know who makes the transition from this life, with a ritual celebration.

There is also a deeper way to honor these teachers, by integrating the lessons they have presented. Through them I have altered my practice and changed my way of being. And no one's lessons have had a more profound impact on me than those of Little Lady, a small bundle of short, chocolate-black fur and a strong voice. She'd been a stray, near-dead with pneumonia, when she was found and rushed to veterinary care. The veterinarian asked if I would help find a home for her, when she recovered.

She had a pile of challenges to overcome: an infection that required an emergency spay to remove a pus-filled uterus and a urinary tract infection. With Reiki, she was able to keep her tongue in her mouth; otherwise it hung out because of neurological damage. With veterinary permission, I gave her Noni juice because it is high in antioxidants, and the bumps that covered her body disappeared. But by then, we knew it would be difficult to find her a home, because blood work had revealed active feline leukemia. Cats with this disease are fragile and can be contagious to others, so she needed to be the only cat in a household. But no one wanted to risk the medical bills and heartbreak that could be part and parcel of such an adoption.

When she began to chafe at the confinement of the clinic's isolation unit, I let her spend weekends in my home, in a room that was fitted with a glass door to keep her from the rest of my cat family. That door was an effective barrier until Kahlua, known for her dexterous paws, figured out how to open it. I woke up one morning to find Little Lady outside her room and Kahlua, inside. Since my other cats had already been exposed to the leukemia virus, I decided that the universe was telling me to make Little Lady a full-fledged family member. (My cats tested negative for the virus and continue to do so.)

Little Lady enjoyed being part of a family and loved the freedom of her expanded world. She developed a healthy coat. Her eyes were bright and her energy level high. To supplement conventional care, she took herbal remedies and had acupuncture treatments that helped control many of her symptoms. She was doing so well that I gave her *distance* at less regular intervals. She still received *hands on* though, for shorter periods than before. I forgot my past experience with leukemia cats; just like kidney cats, cutting back on Reiki can have sudden and tragic consequences.

I'd had a funny feeling for a couple of weeks that something was wrong, but I couldn't put my finger on it. There was no evidence to warrant a veterinary visit, so I held off until her regular appointment. Then things took a turn for the worse. She started to vomit and couldn't stop. She was anemic and both her red and white blood

counts were low. Hours after she started to turn around with veterinary intervention, the problem would start again. When she seemed to have stabilized, she was released to my care.

In the early hours of the following morning, I knew I was losing her, but I had no money to pay for off-hour emergency care. So I shared *hands on* with her continuously - a profoundly spiritual experience permeated with deep peace and acceptance of the inevitable. While I felt that I should just let nature take its course, a quick chat with the veterinarian gave me the hope that changed my mind. So, I took her to the clinic and after massive intervention, she died, waiting for a blood transfusion, at less than two years old.

I've reflected on my actions during those last four days of hell. I made mistakes, the same ones I'd often chastised others for: ignoring premonitions because of a lack of hard evidence; deferring to authority under stress; reverting under pressure to the automatic pilot of old ways of being, thus limiting my options; failing to appreciate the implications of seemingly helpful actions I'd made before, that limited my ability to respond to her when she needed it most. And after intensive reflection, I acknowledged that I wasn't the only one who'd made mistakes, and that I needed to change.

For someone who is guided so much by bodily sensations, it may be hard to understand how I could have ignored those vague feelings about Little Lady in my gut. Thanks to her, I honored those premonitions with Friend (as I described in Chapter Eight), a few months after Little Lady died. On the flimsiest of evidence, I took her to the veterinarian, only to find that her kidneys were starting to become inflamed. I have no regrets for intervening so early in the process. I have no doubt that it has been life-extending, if not life-saving, for Friend.

Too often during those four days of hell, I set aside my gut instincts, not wanting to hurt the feelings of others or upset their schedules and practices. I had my chance to do it differently with Cathryn Twinkletoes when she had a stroke. Her person called the veterinary clinic only to be told that she should wait for an hour or so until the veterinarian could speak with her, before bringing the cat in. She called me to ask for Reiki and I immediately turned my car around, picked her up, and told her to call the clinic on my cell

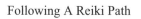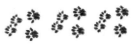

phone. "Tell them," I said in my new, feisty voice, "that we're coming in, so don't close the doors. If after they see her they want us to leave, we will. But not until then." One look at Cathryn and it was an acknowledged veterinary emergency. We have Little Lady to thank for taking action rather than politely waiting, afraid to rock the boat.

Like many of those in the helping professions, I'd put my needs and those of my immediate family on the back burner, to answer another's call for help. I didn't act on my vague feelings about Little Lady partly because of a lack of hard evidence, and partly because I was so busy twisting myself out of shape to meet the constant demands of two of my most manipulative clients, people who used fake pet emergencies to lure me into providing them with constant attention.

I cannot change the way people behave, but I have since examined my actions. And I'm far less inclined to distort my priorities at the demand of a needy person who is likely to cry wolf. Some people use their pets as an excuse to get attention, taking time away from a Reiki session with discussions of their traumas and needs. Now, I am more able to clearly tell them that they need to meet those needs in another way; because one thing is certain: I am there for the pet, not the pet's person. And if they deny me access to that pet, by taking up my time with their tales of woe or requests for other services, I walk out the door.

Similarly, I have set clearer financial boundaries. One of the things I regret was my inability to get emergency care for Little Lady because I had no funds. My credit card was maxed out from paying the bills for some clients' pet care, clients who I later found out could well have afforded to pay their bills and reimburse me promptly. Since then, I've limited my financial sponsorship to a pet whose person is on welfare.

I continue to respect Little Lady and what she stands for, by refining my practice of this stronger set of life rules: to be guided by gut as much as fact, to assert the needs of my pet even if it may inconvenience others, and to adhere to stronger emotional and financial boundaries. I'd love to say that my implementation is

131

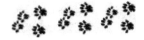

totally flawless and consistent, but I am still on a steep learning curve. Grief has ripped a hole in my heart where her memory lives forever, but I cannot bear the thought that she died in vain. So instead, I work on my practice of the many lessons she taught me. That is how I adhere to the Reiki precept, by honoring one of the greatest teachers I've ever had.

Kindness.
Treat everything that lives with good will and generosity.

The fifth Reiki precept is about kindness, treating everything that lives with good will and generosity. There is no better opportunity to show kindness than in the face of suffering. And that is the chance we get with an ailing or dying pet. When pets' bodies are at their weakest, as energy levels decrease, appetites wane, and problems with grooming and toileting come to the fore, we can offer comfort and support. This has little to do with whether or not you use *hands on* or *distance* and everything with Reiki's intent to show loving kindness to every living being.

Many pets have given me the opportunity to learn this Reiki precept and one of the best such teachers is Seraphim, a sweet cat suffering the ravages of old age. While she is well-loved, her people are sometimes too distressed by the deterioration they witness to provide anything but the most rudimentary care. Yet, they are unwilling to let her go. And as importantly, Seraphim shows a strong will to live, maintaining her interest in food, her use of the litter box, and her monitoring of birds.

Most of my visits to her are when her people are at work. This gives me the chance to offer some tender loving care in addition to Reiki and because of this, our sessions usually last two hours instead of one. If she is having a bad day, she often hunches up (a sure sign of pain) and if she is in that position with her neck outstretched, I know she is nauseous. So I direct *distance* to her nausea before offering her anything to eat.

Sooner or later, I get down to the business of food. On her bad days, Seraphim upsets her people when she refuses to eat. And keeping a sick cat interested in food can be critical; for the absence

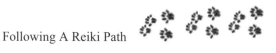

of adequate food can lead to compromised liver function, a condition that is extremely difficult to reverse (except at the earliest stages) and often leads to death. As a former chef, I know how to make her food appealing, which means that it is fresh and served in a clean dish; and if it is wet food, I serve it at room temperature or slightly warmer (by zapping it in a microwave or heating it over a bowl of warm water). This also releases the smell of the food which can be an appetite stimulant. Because she will only eat small amounts, I offer her a high-calorie food supplement (with veterinary permission) in addition to her prescription food or homemade diet. There are days when she decides she is on a diet and just won't eat. Then, I resort to her old-time favorite, Heinz baby food chicken. While I'm not in the habit of endorsing particular brands, this is the only one in my area which has no salt, herbs, spices, vegetables, flavorings, or additives that could upset her stomach or cause further medical problems.

When she has gotten to the baby food stage, she is often too tired or weak to eat, so I spoon feed her. And, on those days when spoon feeding is refused, she gets force fed using a medium-sized syringe (without the needle) filled with creamy wet food and inserted into the side of her mouth. A normal meal that may be eaten in a matter of minutes, now takes an hour to consume. This gives me an opportunity to practise patience. I keep focused on the present, praising her with every mouthful she eats.

As her body ages, she becomes dehydrated more frequently. Dehydration curbs her appetite even more and makes her body ache. To keep her hydrated, I thin her wet food slightly with water. And to supplement her water intake, since cats are notorious for not drinking enough, I make her Smudge's chicken latte (named for a cat who adores this recipe) or homemade chicken soup.

<u>Smudge's Chicken Latte</u>
- 1 teaspoon of chicken baby food (chicken and broth only with nothing added; no salt, herbs, spices, flavorings. Check the label, Heinz is one such brand).

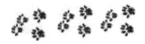

- 1/8 to 1/4 cup water at room temperature, preferably filtered.
- Mix together in a bowl and present to the pet.

Susan's Chicken Broth for Pets
- Chicken necks and backs.
- Cold water.
- Put chicken necks and backs into a pot with enough cold water to cover them completely. Bring this mixture to a boil.
- As soon as the mixture is boiling, reduce the heat to a slow boil. Leave the pot uncovered, cooking the liquid until it has been reduced by half.
- Remove the carcass and bones and throw them out because they no longer have any nutritional value. You may find it easier to remove them out by pouring the mixture into a strainer lined with a few layers of cheesecloth - just don't forget to put the strainer over a bowl.
- Put the liquid in a covered container and refrigerate. Fat will solidify on the top. Remove it with a spoon and discard it.
- To serve, take out the amount you need and warm it slightly. If you put a drop of it against the inside of your wrist it should feel comfortably warm. Make sure it is not too warm. Then put the liquid in a pet dish, or spoon or syringe (without the needle) into the pet's mouth.

I check her hydration by pulling up the skin between her shoulder blades and letting it fall. The longer it takes to fall, the more hydration she needs. When she lets me, I run my finger along her gums. When they are sticky, she needs to be hydrated. Her people have been trained by their veterinarian to give subcutaneous hydration, where what looks like an intravenous needle is inserted between the shoulders just under the skin and fluids are given. Because she wriggles away during this process, she is placed in a

134

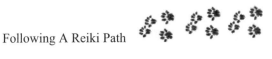

restraint bag which calms her because she is enclosed from the neck down.

Like many clients, her people are leery about giving her medications, yet administering them properly and on schedule can be critical. Sometimes, they resort to mixing them into food in the hopes that the she will consume them. If the medications are tasteless or minimally awful, she will comply. But if the medicine is vile-tasting, I mix it with water and put it in a syringe without a needle and then into the side of her mouth. That way, the medication does not turn her off her food. She seems to understand when I give her vile-tasting medicine or have to force feed, that I am doing this with the best of intentions. And she accepts. Inevitably, some food or medicine spilled on her fur needs to be wiped clean with a warm washcloth.

When dinner is over, I refill her bowl with fresh, filtered water and change the towels over her bedding. I brought a soft foam pad to put under her towel to cushion her fragile body. And Santa gave her a heat-reflector pad that soothes her sore joints. I clean her litter box, checking for hard, round stools, a sure sign of constipation and the need to either use a laxative or add more water and fiber to her meals. Only after we have completed these tasks is she truly ready for Reiki.

I cannot stop Seraphim from aging and I cannot make everything better. But in small ways, I can make her day just a little more comfortable and pleasant. These simple chores remind me that ordinary moments are precious because they make up the bulk of our interactions with pets. And so I focus on doing small things for Seraphim with great love.

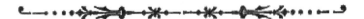

Learning to embody Reiki is a life-long challenge. Goals based on its precepts are eminently reachable and completely elusive. Sometimes I get an intuitive understanding of a precept and feel that it is sitting just right with me, just at that moment. At other times, the

precept is like a mirage, never quite materializing, always eluding my grasp. Just when I think I have mastered it, another lesson comes along that opens that precept back up for deeper, more thorough examination. Like any growth process, it continually unfolds; it is always a matter of becoming.

Chapter 12

Laughing at My Limitations: Lessons in Humility

Kahlua is the mascot of my business, Reiki for Pets. Her stunning photograph graces my brochures and she participates in the teaching of Reiki by volunteering her body for practice. In addition to helping me to teach and my students to learn, Kahlua continues to teach me by being the exception to the rule.

Take her health-style, for example. Most pets will seek Reiki when they are not feeling well. And that is so helpful, especially when there may be a problem that has yet to become obvious. Kahlua is the exception. While still a young senior (age seven years), she has arthritis and a sciatic nerve condition. Both are helped by Reiki *when* I am able to pick up on the cues, but she keeps her physical problems to herself. Ironically, she is more than capable of having an emotional meltdown if I move her food dish, but I have learned the hard way that she could be near death, yet not seek Reiki. Why this is, is a mystery to me.

A while back, I took her to the veterinarian for her annual physical. Her doctor insists on annual blood and urine samples which is fortunate, considering Kahlua's lack of visible cues. It took time to stalk her and get enough urine in the saucer to provide a decent sample. And when it was analyzed, much to both the doctor's and my surprise, Kahlua had a bladder infection! She has never, to my knowledge, had an infection before. She gave me no warning, showing absolutely no change in behavior. Yet, again, she had taken me by surprise.

As a result, she is in the process of teaching me about subtlety. I had thought that as one who has practiced Reiki several times a day for ten years, I completely appreciated the nature of subtlety. After all, Reiki involves the use of subtle energy. Though its impact can be widespread and, at times, hard-hitting, it is usually portrayed as a gentle therapy, channeling a soft, energetic flow through the channel

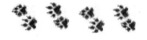

to the receiver. Changes can be great, but just as often they seem to be painstakingly gradual and small. That is what I understand about Reiki.

I always thought cats were the subtlest of beings, using verbal or direct body language only when absolutely necessary. I'm usually able to pick up on small changes in daily behavior patterns: gait, eating, play, sleep, or elimination habits. It has been a source of pride for me to detect something wrong with a pet when others are not aware of it. I thought I'd had ample exposure to enough, different pets to have this down pat. And then along comes Kahlua, who humbles me with ease. Perhaps, she is saving me from becoming too full of pride. But I have enough self-esteem issues that it doesn't take much for me to realize where my areas of incompetence and ignorance lie.

I believe Kahlua is a special teacher for me. She is guiding me to a deeper appreciation of the mysterious relationship between the practitioner and the pet. And like any woman of mystery, her focus is on that which is hidden, obscure, and remains unexplained. I hope that in time, I will either share her secret or fully accept that it is one I will never know. And just as I think I've figured this out to the point of acceptance, Kahlua tosses a new curve into the equation.

Recently, I awoke, aware of a huge Reiki draw from my hands. Kahlua had crawled into bed, positioned her hips under my hands, and was receiving Reiki. I didn't let on that I was awake and the session continued. The next night when this happened, I let her know I was awake. She responded with Siamese profanity to let me know that I was dirtying her fur with my hands and then walked away in a huff. As always, I am humbled in the presence of my teacher. And obviously, I've yet to figure out this new lesson I'm supposed to learn.

If Kahlua could speak English, I'm sure she'd take credit for reinforcing all the lessons I think I have learned about pet-oriented Reiki. She would also take delight in so ably demonstrating the limitations of my learning. I can just hear her say, "It's my job to tease you, so you won't take yourself so seriously. After all, it's not your fault that you are merely human." As I write this, Kahlua is hunched over the sink, licking lemon icing off a plate. "Wait a

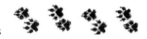

minute," I say to myself. "I put that plate in there knowing cats hate the smell of citrus fruits!" And then I chuckle. Stumped again by Kahlua.

Glossary

Attunement: A way in which a Reiki Master opens up your in-born, though dormant, ability to draw Reiki energy through your body from outside yourself, and direct it toward a being.

Blocking: The ability of a being, who is familiar with Reiki, to divert *distance* being sent to another, to himself. To the best of my knowledge, this appears to happen only with animals.

Calling: Requests for Reiki from a pet, received as sensations specific to that pet.

Channel: A Reiki initiate capable of taking Reiki energy from outside herself and transmitting it through her hands (or feet) to another being.

Directed Reiki: *Distance* Reiki sent to a specific condition, recommended only under certain conditions (see Appendix A).

Distance: Non-contact Reiki, sent with the use of symbols and related mantras.

Draw: A feeling in the channel's body of the intensity of Reiki being taken by the recipient.

Energetic Signature: The means by which a being can recognize or contact another being, energetically. I believe each of us has a distinct energetic signature.

Groundedness: A condition in which a being is fully present in her body, enabling herself to take energy into her body from outside herself and disperse excess energy from her body to the outside. Many humans sense groundedness as a feeling of their feet being strongly connected to the core of the earth. An ungrounded human may have a sense of lightheadedness, of floating outside her body and may experience dizziness, headaches, or a sense of congestion.

Hands On: Contact Reiki, in which the hands of the channel are in direct contact with the body of the recipient.

Healing Attunement: A more intense form of Reiki developed by William Lee Rand. Although it is called an attunement, it is not initiatory. It can be particularly useful for pets who consistently require sessions longer than three hours, but only if they tolerate it. See Appendix A for further details.

Hertz: A measure of frequency or vibration. One Hertz is equivalent to one cycle or vibration per second.

Hitchhiking: The ability of beings in the vicinity where Reiki is being shared to use some of its overflow for themselves.

Initiation: The process of attunement.

Level One: The most basic level of Reiki, at which contact Reiki and self-treatments are taught. For humans, this involves learning specific hand positions.

Level Two: The level at which non-contact Reiki, known as distance, is taught, enabling the initiate to focus her intent with the aid of specific symbols and associated mantras.

Master: A person able to initiate others. Bona fide Masters can trace their lineage back to the discoverer of Reiki, Dr. Usui.

Mastery: Depending upon the Reiki school, this is either a level more advanced than Level Two, or the level of highest initiation which enables a person to initiate others. In some schools, the latter is referred to as Master/Teacher.

mmol/L: Millimoles per liter. In this book, it is associated with BUN (Blood Urea Nitrogen) as a measure of kidney function.

Mental/Emotional Symbol: One of the symbols that can be used with *distance*.

nmol/L: Nanamoles per liter. In this book, it is associated with thyroxine levels, as a measure of thyroid function.

Non-directed Distance Reiki: Reiki sent to a specific being with the understanding that it will go to where it is most needed.

Reiki: A Japanese term for Universal Life Energy given to a method of channeling that energy developed by Dr. Mikao Usui in the mid-1800s and brought to the United States by Hawayo Takata in the 1930s. Since her death in 1980 many schools of Reiki have developed, some of which have added other esoteric teachings.

Reiki Circle: A gathering of people who are Reiki initiates (that is, they have at least Level One) to share Reiki with each other and ask questions of their Master. Most Reiki circles meet on a regular basis (weekly, bimonthly, or monthly). Such meetings are one of the few opportunities that practitioners may have to receive a Reiki session. If the Master attends, meetings also become an opportunity to learn more about Reiki from the responses given to questions posed.

Self-Treatment: A way to take Reiki from outside your body into yourself, for the purpose of treating yourself rather than for sharing it with others.

Session: Sharing Reiki with a being for a period of time. Also called a treatment.

Subcutaneous Hydration: Giving fluids under the skin via a needle, usually attached to a bag of liquids. The best explanation of how to give subcutaneous hydration is in *The New Natural Cat* by Anitra Frazier and Norma Eckroate.

Transmitter: See channel.

Treatment: See session. The word, treatment, had traditionally been used to describe a Reiki session even though Reiki is not a medical practise.

μmol/L: Micromoles per liter. In this book, it is associated with creatinine, as a measure of kidney function.

Appendix A

Applying Pet-Oriented Reiki: A Summary of

Lessons

Each lesson in this Appendix is referenced to the chapter in which it appears.

1. Benefits of Reiki
   a. Behavioral Change
      i. Sending hearts of love through Reiki, supports pets who are sad, timid, insecure, lonely, unwanted, or dying (Chapter 11: Sara).

      ii. In severe behavioral cases, a modest amount of Reiki will have little effect (Chapter 6: Buffalo Bill).

      iii. Anxiety: Reiki can help mitigate anxiety throughout a household (Chapter 6: Mouser).

      iv. Counter-conditioning Anxiety: Reiki can help a pet relax in situations that usually make him uptight (Chapter 6: Mouser).

      v. Self-mutilation: Reiki can help a pet stop self-mutilation that is behaviorally-based. It requires sessions over extended periods to get permanent results, because of the backsliding that is inherent in the ailment (Chapter 6: Geoffrey).

b.   Bond Enhancement: Sharing Reiki can strengthen the human-animal bond. (Chapter 5: Crackle, Christmas Blessing).

c.   Cancer: Reiki is useful in the management of cancer (Chapter 7).

d.   Chemotherapy - Management of Side-Effects: Reiki can best manage the side-effects of chemotherapy when the sessions are started at the time that the chemotherapy session begins (Chapter 7: Samantha).

e.   Diabetes Management: Consistent, regular Reiki can help a pet reduce her insulin requirements. Withdraw the Reiki and the insulin needs climb up again (Chapter 8, Snowball).

f.   Dying and Death: Reiki can help the pet's physical transition at death (Chapter 9:   Midnight, Shiloh, Mugsy, Cathryn Twinkletoes).

g.   Hyperthyroidism Management: Consistent, regular Reiki (specifically, *directed distance*) may reduce bodily stress enough to alter high thyroid levels. Withdraw the Reiki and the levels climb again (Chapter 8, Fuzzy).

h.   Kidney Disease Management: Reiki can normalize the standard parameters for the measurement of kidney disease (BUN and creatinine). Withdraw the Reiki and the measures change back (Chapter 8, Friend).

i.   Nausea Elimination: Reiki is useful for eliminating nausea (Chapter 7, Samantha; Chapter 10: Higgins; Chapter 11, Seraphim).

j.   <u>Pain Management</u>: Reiki can improve a pet's quality of life through the management of short and long-term pain (Chapter 2: Maxine; Chapter 5).

     i.   Reiki is a useful pain management tool, especially in cases where drugs are not effective or cannot be used (Chapter 3; Chapter 5: Blessing; Chapter 11, Ginger).

     ii.   Reiki can help manage acute pain (Chapter 7: Samantha; Chapter 11: Ginger).

     iii.   Reiki can be useful in quieting or eliminating phantom pain (Chapter 6: Sammy).

k.   <u>Palliation of Chronic Illness</u>: Reiki can increase the comfort of old age by palliating the chronic illnesses that often accompany it (Chapter 8; Chapter 11, Seraphim).

l.   <u>Pancreatitis</u>: See 3c, iii in this Appendix.

m.   <u>Releasing Energetic Build-Up in Beings</u>: Reiki can enable a being to release an energetic build-up of emotions (Chapter 6: Geoffrey) or physical debris (Chapter 7: Timmy). Such sessions may have to be extended for the releasing to be completed (Chapter 7: Timmy).

n.   <u>Releasing Energetic Build-Up in Living Space</u>: Reiki can be used to clear space of energetic residual related to pain, trauma, or negative energy (Chapter 9: Cathryn Twinkletoes).

o.   Surgical Recovery: Reiki can aid in a pet's recovery from surgery (Chapter 7: Spiffy, Samantha, Timmy; Chapter 9: Samara).

p.   Soul Care: Reiki can assist the soul both as the pet is dying and after death (Chapter 9: Shiloh, Mugsy, Cathryn Twinkletoes).

q.   Temporomandibular Joint Dysfunction: See 3c, iii in this Appendix.

2.   Diabetes - Special Care: Pets receiving Reiki as palliation for diabetes need a snack immediately following a session. They should also be monitored for the next few hours (Chapter 8, Snowball). See also Benefits of Reiki, 1e in this Appendix.

3.   Forms of Reiki
      a.   General
            A pet's sensitivity to energy varies and thus, also his tolerance for *hands on* or interest in *distance* (Chapter 2).

      b.   *Hands On*
            i.   *Hands on* works best when you can be with the pet in person and the pet is willing and able to be touched (Chapter 3).

            ii.   Save *hands on* until you and the pet are comfortable with each other, even if that takes more than one session to do so (Chapter 2).

            iii.   *Hands on* is more easily accepted when you start by stroking the pet's head and after a time, slowly lower your other palm for direct contact (Chapter 2).

iv.   Pets respond best when *hands on* is delivered without pressure. If need be, float your hand above the area or switch to *distance*, particularly if the area is sensitive (Chapter 2).

v.   Many animals have sensitive rear ends. Approach that area with caution (Chapter 2).

vi.   Don't worry about hand placement. Either the pet will allow you to place your hands where you wish them to go or he will guide you. Respect his wishes (Chapter 2: Tabby, Wye, Kahlua, Friend).

vii.   The Reiki hand positions for humans often do not apply when working with pets. Some positions, such as placing your hands over the eyes, can frighten non-human beings (Chapter 1; Chapter 2).

c.   <u>Distance</u>

i.   *Distance* Reiki has a number of uses: as an introduction before an in-person meeting or a way of keeping in touch between meetings; in an emergency; when the pet cannot be directly touched because of pain or an open wound or infection; with animals who cannot tolerate touch because of anxiety or emotional problems; and when you are at risk from physical harm (Chapter 3).

ii.   Situations in which the pet is uncomfortable with or new to Reiki, are best started with *distance* (Chapter 2).

149

iii. *Distance directed* to a specific *condition* is helpful in the following four situations: nausea (Chapter 7, Samantha; Chapter10:Higgins), temporomandibular joint pain (Chapter 5: Blessing), hyperthyroidism (Chapter 8: Fuzzy), and pancreatitis (Chapter 10: Higgins). Direct the Reiki to the condition rather than to a specific organ or disease (e.g., to the nausea condition, not to the nausea) so it takes care of the totality of the problem. However, if *directed distance* is used extensively, you must ensure that an equal or greater amount of *non-directed Reiki* is also provided to look after the pet's overall wellness (Chapter 3; Chapter 10: Higgins).

iv. If the situation is complex or not responding to Reiki, request that the Reiki go to the core problem of that entire condition, rather than to a specific ailment or organ (Chapter 10: Higgins).

d. Healing Attunement
i. Healing attunements work well with terminally and chronically ill pets if they can tolerate them. Such pets have need of more than three hours of Reiki a day (Chapter 7: Timmy; Chapter 8: Friend; Chapter 11). Use caution with frail and elderly pets (Chapter 8: Penny).

ii. It is important to be physically present at the first few healing attunements to monitor the pet's reaction to them. If the pet becomes frightened or upset after receiving a healing attunement, such attunements should be discontinued (Chapter 3).

150

4.   First Session

    a.   First sessions take longer because of the need for introductions. My rule of thumb is that a typical session is 60 minutes, but a first session is 90 (Chapter 2).

    b.   When meeting a pet for the first time, take your time with introductions. If possible, let the pet come to you (Chapter 2).

    c.   A skittish or apprehensive pet may be helped by the presence of his person, especially if that person is relaxed and can stroke him or sit beside him during his first session (Chapter 2: Maxine).

5.   Is The Pet Ready to Die? Just because an animal is failing, doesn't mean he wants to die. Lethargy and lack of appetite may be signs of ill health and nothing more. If the pet accepts force feeding, it is an indicator of wish to live (Chapter 9, Samara). Others include the ability to maintain toilet habits, continued ability to groom (cats), and interest in one's surroundings (Chapter 11, Seraphim).

6.   Preparing for the Session

    a.   If possible, send *distance* to a pet before your first meeting so he can recognize your energetic signature when you meet in person (Chapter 2).

    b.   Before you meet him, find out as much as you can about the pet and his situation. Consider what this might mean for how to approach him or how to structure the session (Chapter 2).

    c.   Learn about animal behavior to know appropriate greeting rituals, idiosyncrasies of particular species and breeds, and what behavior is normal (Appendix

D). Consider what this might mean for how to approach a pet or how to structure the session (Chapter 2).

7. Reducing or Stopping Reiki

a. Pets who do not want Reiki (or are finished with the session) will remove themselves from your hands or break the *distance* connection. Some will swat hands away or nip (Chapter 2). If the pet pulls away or growls during an otherwise peaceful session, this is a signal to end the session (Chapter 3). See also 14c in this Appendix.

b. Chronically ill and terminally ill pets can experience a health crisis if Reiki is decreased or discontinued (Chapter 4; Chapter 8: Friend; Chapter 11: Ginger; Little Lady).

c. If a person has been advised by another professional to cut back on Reiki, it is important to prevent a relapse. Decrease the sessions slowly and observe the effect rather than stopping them all at once (if the person is willing to try this) (Chapter 4).

8. Reiki Practice

a. The best way for a practitioner to ensure that Reiki is clearly transmitted, is through regular self-treatments (Chapter 3; Chapter 11).

b. Pets who need large amounts of Reiki tend to have a strong draw. In such circumstances, the sender must stay grounded so that she won't be affected by that draw (Chapter 7; Chapter 10: Miss Demeanor).

c. Reiki can be safely shared with pets under anesthetic (Chapter 10: Beakers).

d. A pet's person's decisions about euthanasia are one of the most challenging areas in which the practitioner is called to set judgment aside (Chapter 9: Shiloh, Mugsy).

e. Those for whom you have the greatest responsibility are yourself and your immediate family, regardless of the needs of others (Chapter 11: Little Lady).

f. Sometimes it's okay to rock the boat (Chapter 11: Little Lady).

g. There is always another lesson to learn (Chapter 12: Kahlua).

h. There is always an exception to every rule of thumb I have developed (Chapter 12).

i. It is useful to test every assumption about Reiki yourself (Chapter 10).

j. It takes a long time to develop a viable, full-time Reiki practice (Chapter 11; Appendix D).

k. The spirit of Reiki is transmitted by kindness (Chapter 11, Seraphim).

l. Information from sharing Reiki with a pet may be useful to other professionals in assessing that pet, monitoring his progress, or changing treatment protocols (Chapter 4).

m. Hygiene Matters
    i. Learn about precautionary measures to prevent the spread of contagious diseases to other pets (Chapter 11; Appendix D).

ii. Minimize the risk from working with ill pets, to yourself and your own pets (Appendix D).

iii. Wash your hands before and after working with each pet, to prevent spread of germs (Chapter 2; Appendix D).

iv. Be careful not to touch an open wound or sore. Float your hands over the area instead (Chapter 2).

v. Keep a change of clothing nearby in case a pet soils your clothes (Chapter 2).

9. <u>Reiki Relationship: Practitioner and Pet</u>

a. Pets are active participants in Reiki (Chapter 2; Chapter 3).

b. Fundamental to the spirit of Reiki is the concept of consent. Thus it is important to have the pet's consent for Reiki (Chapter 2), for attunement to Reiki (Chapter 10), and for continued life or euthanasia (Chapter 9).

c. Taking the time to establish a safe Reiki relationship, ensures that the pet's participation is based on willingness and trust (Chapter 2).

d. Let the pet have as much control as possible over the timing, location, and acceptance of Reiki (Chapter 2).

i. Pets are most receptive to Reiki during their quiet times.

ii. Pets are more relaxed and receptive to Reiki if the session is held in a location they favor.

154

iii.   Slowly introducing a pet to Reiki gives him a chance to get used to it and increases the chances of his acceptance of it (Chapter 2).

e.   Staying calm, talking softly, and breathing slowly can help a nervous pet to relax (Chapter 2).

f.   When a pet refuses to accept Reiki, that refusal needs to be honored (Chapter 2: Smoky).

g.   It's possible to accommodate the pet by modifying your behavior based on her verbal and non-verbal signals. For example, if she is uncomfortable with two hands, switch to one; if she is uncomfortable with *hands on*, switch to *distance* (Chapter 2).

h.   Many animals prefer the contact of one hand rather than two (Chapter 2).

i.   Hovering your hands over sensitive areas is better received than using direct contact (Chapter 2).

j.   Sometimes a pet will direct you to the part of the body that is most affected (Chapter 7: Samantha). A pet's asking for Reiki, especially in a particular area, may signal the onset of health problems (Chapter 5: Blessing; Chapter 8: Friend).

k.   A pet can energetically request Reiki once she has been introduced to it (Chapter 3).

i.   Interruptions or energetic calls for Reiki can manifest as sensations in the practitioner's body, affecting any one of the sensory systems (Chapter 3).

ii. Some pets are patient enough to call and then wait until you can share Reiki with them. Some have no patience and divert Reiki immediately (Chapter 3).

iii. Interruptions or energetic calls for Reiki can come from more than one pet at the same time (Chapter 3).

l. *Distance* sessions can be interrupted or diverted. A pet who has received intensive Reiki sessions is capable of diverting other *distance* sessions to himself (Chapter 3: Ginger, Blessing).

    i. A pet in dire need can divert all *distance* Reiki sent by the person he is calling, to himself (Chapter 3: Ginger, Blessing).

    ii. Diverting Reiki is not influenced by the intent of the sender or the size of the receiver (Chapter 3).

    iii. Pets seem to be able to teach other pets in the household to divert Reiki as well (Chapter 3: Ginger).

m. Pets can direct the course of receiving Reiki by *distance*; some can direct more than one therapy to themselves at the same time (Chapter 3, Beakers).

n. Pets can be attuned to Reiki, though it is preferable to ensure their consent first (Chapter 10: Kahlua, Friend, Christmas Blessing, Timmy, Beauty).

10. Reiki Relationship: Practitioner and the Pet's Person
    a. Make sure you understand the person's expectations of Reiki and that these are achievable, before accepting the appointment (Chapter 2); otherwise,

the person may be disappointed (Chapter 6, Muggins).

b. Keeping track of the pet's changes over time is useful when clients question Reiki's effectiveness. When a pet makes positive changes, it is easy for her person to forget the pet's original condition (Chapter 6, Muggins).

c. The pet's person is often the conduit amongst the various professionals working with her pet (Chapter 4).

d. It is important to establish clear emotional and financial boundaries with the pet's people (Chapter 4; Chapter 11, Little Lady).

e. Some people are pressured by other family members or friends to give up on Reiki and that can influence their willingness to continue with sessions (Chapter 4).

f. Bonds between pets and their humans vary even within the same household, so it is not unusual for one pet to receive treatment and another to be ignored (Chapter 4).

g. When a person is co-dependent with his pet, his own emotional needs can interfere with what is in the pet's best interests (Chapter 4; Chapter 9: Shiloh, Mugsy).

11. Remission - Special Care: Remission does not mean cure. It just means the illness can no longer be detected by conventional means. To reduce Reiki under these circumstances invites a health crisis (Chapter 8: Friend, Simon).

12. <u>Session Follow-Up</u>
    i.   Having the pet's photograph helps focus a *distance* session, especially such sessions sent from outside the pet's home (Chapter 2).

13. <u>Sharing Reiki With More Than One Being At The Same Time</u>
    i.   When sharing Reiki between two beings at once, the flow is divided. The larger portion goes to the being in greatest need (Chapter 3).

    ii.   People and pets can receive some of the benefits of a Reiki session just by being in the same room in which Reiki is being shared (Chapter 3).

    iii.   Other pets in the household may want Reiki regardless of whether or not such provisions have been made. In such cases, a short session will do a lot to alleviate jealousy (Chapter 2).

    iv.   In some cases, it may be best to share Reiki with all interested pets in a household at the same time, using your hands and feet to contact all the bodies involved (Chapter 3).

    v.   Sharing Reiki with fish often requires sharing with the whole school, so that one fish is not singled out (Chapter 2).

14. <u>Time</u>
    a.   Session length is discussed in 4a of this Appendix.

    b.   Length of the session is determined by need, not size (Chapter 10: Miss Demeanor).

    c.   Pets are capable of sharing Reiki for an hour or more. If a pet leaves after a shorter period, he may be asking for a break to assimilate energy rather than announcing that the session is over. Allow the break and then resume. If he then leaves, growls, swats, or nips, it means the session is over (Chapter 2).

d.   As long as the pet is grounded, extensive sessions will not result in energetic overload. An ungrounded pet can be helped by sharing Reiki with her paws (Chapter 3).

e.   Pets with chronic or terminal illness can take a lot of Reiki (Chapter 8: Friend; Chapter 11, Ginger). Even those in acute situations, like recovery from surgery, can require more than an hour at a time (Chapter 7: Samantha).

f.   To help determine if a pet wishes to end a session, see 7a in this Appendix.

g.   Ideally, it is useful to start with Reiki sessions four days in a row, followed by sessions two or three times a week and then slowly decrease the frequency over time (Chapter 6).

h.   Sharing Reiki can alter the perception of time (Chapter 8: Simon).

i.   Reiki seems to alter the time frame within which cancer operates (Chapter 7: Timmy).

j.   Sometimes, persisting with Reiki and even increasing it in the face of negative results can be beneficial (Chapter 8: Simon).

k.   Keeping present-centred enhances the human-pet bond (Chapter 11: Ginger).

l.   Premonitions deserve to be honored (Chapter 4: Gottfreid; Chapter 8: Simon; Chapter 10: Higgins; Chapter 11, Little Lady, Friend).

m.   See also 10b in this Appendix.

15.   <u>Water</u>
Ensure the pet has access to a fresh supply of water to flush the toxins that Reiki can release. With long or frequently repeated Reiki sessions, check the pet's hydration level (Chapter 2; Chapter 10: Higgins).

16.   <u>When The Pet's Person Shares Reiki</u>
a.   Pets who have high Reiki needs (e.g., because of terminal or chronic illness) benefit from receiving regular Reiki sessions from their people (Chapters 4, 6, 8).

b.   Sometimes Reiki requirements are so great that they can best be met by the pet's person and others, supplemented by practitioner sessions (Chapter 7: Timmy).

c.   Having the pet's person learn and share Reiki is one way of reducing the session costs (Chapter 4).

d.   Sharing Reiki is best done when both parties are relaxed and settled. If a pet's person wishes to share Reiki but has difficulty relaxing, the best time for sharing is during a self-treatment session. Otherwise, the pet is better off receiving Reiki from a third party (Chapter 2).

e.   Not all people who share Reiki have the ability to do so on a consistent basis (Chapter 4). If a pet's person is unwilling or unable to share Reiki on a consistent basis and the pet has a chronic illness, the pet is better off receiving Reiki from a third party (Chapter 8: Snowball).

Appendix B

Engaging A Reiki Practitioner or Teacher

Some of you may be interested in trying Reiki for your pet, either by hiring a practitioner or learning how to do it yourself. Here are some suggestions for assessing a suitable practitioner.

Assessing A Practitioner for Your Pet

1.   Think about what you would like in a practitioner for your pet. With what kind of person would you and your pet be most comfortable? Is it important that the person have experience with pets or a particular species, or would a human-oriented practitioner be acceptable? Do you want someone who can visit your home or do you prefer to take your pet elsewhere? What fees are you willing to pay?

2.   Once you know your criteria for hiring such a person, do some research into the resources in your area. If you are not familiar with the different schools of Reiki whose students might be available to you, then consult the community bulletin boards at your local health food or alternative care facility, search the Internet, or read up on Reiki. *The Reiki Sourcebook* by Bronwen and Frans Stiene is one such resource. Ask your friends and other pet lovers for referrals.

3.   Interview potential candidates using the criteria you have developed. Is the practitioner familiar with the kind of problem your pet is experiencing? If you are comfortable with that person, invite her to meet your pet and observe how they interact. By now, you probably know the degree to which the person meets your needs. So, now the two most important things to assess are the level of comfort your pet

and you have with this practitioner, and the results of any references the practitioner provides.

4.   Make sure both of you clearly understand your expectations. Then assess the outcomes of each session. Keep a log with your pet's usual behaviors and condition before Reiki and write up any changes you observe on a daily basis, for at least the first few sessions. Then re-assess your pet's and your comfort with the person and the work that is being done.

5.   Trust your assessment (the results you observed as well as how you feel about the situation). If the outcomes are to your satisfaction but finances are an issue, consider becoming a Reiki student yourself.

6.   Your pet and you need to be able to trust the person with whom you are dealing and believe that she is committed to helping the two of you. If you are not satisfied or feel uncomfortable, look elsewhere. Or, consider becoming a Reiki student so you can care for your pet's energetic needs yourself.

Assessing a Reiki Master In Order to Learn Reiki

1.   Before you approach any Reiki Master, be clear on your reason for wanting to learn Reiki. Are you interested mainly in self-treatment? Are you interested in working with your pet(s) and/or family members? Are your interested in becoming a practitioner?

2.   Figure out which school of Reiki attracts you the most. Consult the resources on the Internet or a book such as *The Reiki Sourcebook* by Bronwen and Frans Stiene for information and ideas. One of the largest differences amongst Reiki schools is the number of attunements given to the initiate at Level One. Some schools do four and others,

one. I believe that the four-attunement initiation process protects the transmitter from sharing the receiver's energetic debris at the physical, emotional, mental, and spiritual levels. Based on your research, you should be able to track down which practitioners of that school live nearest to you.

3. Assess your learning style. Are you comfortable with an intense course where everything is learned over one day or a weekend, or do you prefer a slower pace in order to assimilate new information? The Level One course can range from one, eight-hour day to two-hour sessions for four weeks. For example, some Masters offer a two and a half day weekend course, with the Friday evening as a free session after which you can decide whether or not to continue. Although I will teach in this format as well, I prefer to teach a customized, one-person class over four weeks, giving the student one attunement per week and the opportunity to practise between teaching sessions. Similar timeframes and issues apply to Level Two.

4. Consider the resources you have and your level of need. What are your time and financial constraints? Do you need to learn Reiki quickly because your pet is ill, or can you take your time? Do you need to learn *distance* (Level Two) as soon as possible, because your pet will not accept *hands on* (Level One)?

5. How long an interval needs to pass between learning Level One and Level Two? Some Masters allow you to take both levels in immediate sequence, even on the same weekend. Some insist that you practise Level One for about six months before they will consider you for Level Two.

6. What experience does the Master have with pets? Many Masters have limited experience with non-human animals. In such cases, you will have to adapt what you learn about humans to then apply it to pets.

165

7. It is unusual to be able to transfer your learning between schools, although you can change Masters within the same school. If you take Level One with one school and decide to learn Level Two from a Master of a different school, that Master may require you to re-do your Level One. This is because different schools have different practices. Keep in mind that costs vary; different symbols may be used; there are variations in the number of attunements given at each level; and each school and Master has a particular teaching style.

9. What opportunities are there to hone your Reiki practice? Will the Master be available to you if you have questions after the course? Is there a Reiki circle you can join?

10. Again, once you have figured out your criteria, set up a meeting with the Master(s) in whom you have an interest. Make your selection based not only on the degree to which the person meets your criteria, but also on the depth of rapport and level of comfort you feel with him. Working with a Master can be a long-term engagement, so if your intuition suggests that you should be wary, trust it and move on to someone else.

Appendix C

Using Psychic Spray and Cleanser

Psychic Spray

This formula is intended to cleanse negative energies from home and work spaces. It is adapted from two formulas taught by the Flower Essence Society. I confirmed the value of spray when I took my cat, Kahlua, for a veterinary examination. All the clinic rooms were filled and we were put into the space where euthanasias were conducted. Kahlua became agitated so I whipped out my Psychic Spray bottle and doused the room. When the veterinarian entered, she remarked that something in the room had changed, and it had. The negative energies released in pain and fear had dispersed.

Materials
- A 6 oz. spray bottle, preferably glass.
- Vodka as a preservative (an ounce or so). If you plan to use up the spray more quickly or can't stand the smell of the vodka, just refrigerate the combination instead; refrigerated, it should last up to one week.
- Non-carbonated spring water.
- The following FES Quintessential flower essences* (available in 1/4 oz. stock size).
  Make sure you get flower essences and NOT essential oils.
  Angelica (*angelica archangelica*) to provide a sense of spiritual protection.
  Garlic (*allium sativum*) to strengthen the auric field.
  Mountain Pennyroyal (*monardella odoratissma*) to repel psychic possession or contamination.
  Pink Yarrow (*achillea millefolium var. rubra*) to provide a protective shield for those who tend to absorb others' emotional states.

Shooting Star (*dodecatheon hendersonii*) for groundedness.
Sagebrush (artemesia tridentata) to get rid of that which no longer serves.
Yarrow (achillea millefolium) to provide a protective shield from psychic toxicity and the absorption of negative influences.

Preparation

Pour about 1 oz. of vodka into the spray bottle. It should take up between 1/8 to 1/4 bottle of a 6 oz. bottle; 1/8 will keep the mixture intact for 4 weeks, 1/4 for 8 weeks.

Add sufficient spring water to reach the shoulder of the bottle (where it curves to make a neck).

Add 3 drops of each of the flower essences.

Cover the bottle with the cap and shake it very gently about 12 times.

How to Use

Each time before you use it, shake the bottle gently 6 times or so. Spray throughout a room or space, especially in places like corners where energy can become trapped. You can spray around yourself or your clothes, too.

Psychic Cleanser

This formula is intended to get rid of negative energies, specifically by energetically preparing a space for activities related to deep transformation (e.g., traumatic intervention and/or euthanasia), and by energetically cleansing a space to remove negative energies that could affect beings who enter the room. It is intended for use in veterinary clinics and animal shelters.

Materials

- A 6 oz. spray bottle, preferably glass.
- Vodka as a preservative (an ounce or so). If you plan to use up the spray more quickly or can't stand the smell of the vodka, just refrigerate the combination instead; refrigerated, it should last up to one week.

168

- Non-carbonated spring water.
- The following FES Quintessential flower essences* (available in 1/4 oz. stock size).
Make sure you get flower essences and NOT essential oils.

Angelica (*angelica archangelica*) to provide a sense of spiritual protection.

Angel's Trumpet (*datura candida*) to facilitate surrender or deep transformation.

Garlic (*allium sativum*) to strengthen the auric field.

Mountain Pennyroyal (*monardella odoratissma*) to repel psychic possession or contamination.

Pink Yarrow (*achillea millefolium var. rubra*) to provide a protective shield for those who tend to absorb others' emotional states.

Yarrow (*achillea millefolium*) to provide a protective shield from psychic toxicity and the absorption of negative influences.

Five-Flower Formula™ (also known as Rescue Remedy, consisting of Cherry Plum, Clematis, Impatiens, Rock Rose, and Star of Bethlehem) to ground and centre those in shock or dealing with trauma.

Preparation
The same as for Psychic Spray with the following change. Add 3 drops of each flower essence except for Five-Flower Formula™. Add 6 drops of Five-Flower Formula™.

How to Use
The same as for Psychic Spray.

* Flower essences are available from some health food, new age, and organic grocery stores. For information on local suppliers of FES Quintessentials and English Healing Herbs flower essences, consult www.fesflowers.com

Appendix D

Developing A Pet-Oriented Reiki Practice

I often receive phone calls from aspiring pet practitioners asking for advice on starting a Reiki practice. In my experience, making a livelihood through Reiki stretches one to come to terms with what it means to earn a living with honesty, that is, in a fair and just manner. It results in a lot of soul searching on such issues as running a business, money, veterinary medicine, and death. Here are ten guidelines I ask them to consider.

1. Reiki may be a vocation, but if you accept payment, it is a business, at least for tax purposes. Follow the guidelines for any small business, including getting a bookkeeper or accountant, and obtaining and renewing the necessary licenses for the jurisdiction in which you practise.

2. Decide about the type of business you want: an outcall practice where you travel to the pets' homes or a home-based practice where they come to you. Consider the implications: the costs of transportation and communication if you opt to travel, the effect on your own pets and your neighbours if you receive clients at home.

3. Decide on the kind of pet clientele you will treat. Are you comfortable with cats but not dogs, birds but not turtles? What will you do when you get a call about a pet boa constrictor or the local zoo contacts you about an elephant? Will you restrict your clientele to those living in the better parts of the community or are you willing to enter the seedy side of town?

171

4. Put safety first. Discuss with a veterinarian the precautions you need to take so you don't spread disease from one house to the next. Learn how to wash your hands properly; the local public health authority can provide information on how to do this. Also, discuss the need for vaccinations for your own pets because of the potential risks to them. Find out what vaccinations you should receive (likely the same ones taken by veterinary staff) to provide immunity to rabies, and prevent infections from bites and scratches. Some of you may prefer not to proceed with vaccinations based on a philosophy of natural care. Still, it is worthwhile discussing risk minimization with your veterinarian.

5. Consider the prices you charge, because they affect both your ability to earn a living and the kinds of pets you can have as clients. Under what circumstances will you give discounts? Free treatment? What will you do when the pet is responding well to Reiki but the people cannot afford to continue with the sessions? What will you do when you are working with an animal who is in dire need of veterinary treatment his people cannot afford?

6. Read about or take courses on animal behavior so you have a better understanding of the pets with whom you deal. Learn the signals they give you that say they are afraid, nervous, fearful, ready to attack, defensive, or in pain. Learn how to diffuse potentially difficult situations. Accept the fact that you will get bitten, scratched, vomited, urinated, and defecated on at least sometimes in your practice. So, make sure you have had your shots (if you had decided to proceed with them), and have a first aid kit and a spare change of clothing available at all times.

7. Learn the signs of a veterinary emergency. Some caregivers will prefer using you to a veterinarian, but it is against the law for you to offer veterinary advice or to allow an animal to remain in distress. You can, however, suggest people get a second opinion if the treatment they are pursuing for their

pet doesn't appear to be effective. Keep in mind that some behavioral problems are really medical (for example, housesoiling can be a sign of a urinary tract infection) and can be life-threatening if untreated. Learn about the anatomy of those species you work with. It can help you express your findings more clearly to others. Just don't expect Reiki to solve a veterinary problem. It may help, but it can't cure.

8. Decide whether or not you will take clients who require euthanasia. Reflect on your own views of assisted and non-assisted death. Will you provide Reiki to a pet during euthanasia? Will you take the pet to a clinic to be euthanized in the person's stead? What will you do if you believe the pet does not want to die but the person insists on it? If the pet is ready to die, but the person will not let go? What kinds of support are you willing to offer a grieving household?

9. It takes a long time and a lot of effort to develop a Reiki practice. Be prepared to have another source of dependable income until the practice is viable; that may take years.

10. Remember that self-treatment is the basis of Reiki. Make sure you allow yourself time for regular sessions.

Addressing these issues is an ongoing process that stretches your comfort zone and forces you to confront your values and attitudes, often at the most unexpected times. And that is part of the challenge of pet-oriented Reiki.

References

Anitra Frazier, A. with Eckroat, N. 1990. *The new natural cat: A complete guide for finicky owners.* 3rd Edition. New York: Plume.

Stiene, B. and Stiene, F. 2003. *The Reiki sourcebook.* New York: O Books.

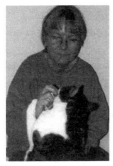

About the Authors

Susan Mack trained as a professional chef, and owned and operated Wine and Roses, a restaurant in Edmonton, Canada. Following a serious illness, she tried Reiki and became so impressed with its ability to heal that she became a Reiki student (Usui Shiki Ryoho). Immediately, the cats and dogs of family and friends started putting themselves under her hands to receive the healing energy. So at their recommendation, she started Reiki for Pets™, an outcall practice exclusively serving pets and their people since 1994. Each year she provides over 2,000 Reiki sessions, continually learning from the pets themselves. She became a Reiki Master/Teacher in 2000 (Traditional Japanese Reiki). She continues her practice as an independent Master, unaffiliated with any Reiki school.

As a Reiki Teacher, Susan accepts students interested in working with their own pets. She conducts individualized courses, often in the pet's home. She also taught a pet-oriented Reiki class in the Continuing Education Division of Edmonton Public Schools.

Susan has written a column on pets for the Reiki Practitioners' Association Newsletter since that column's inception in 1995 until 2006. Her work has been featured on local and national television, radio, newspapers and magazines. For example, she made the front-page feature of the Living Section of the Edmonton Journal (1997). She was the first pet-oriented practitioner to be the subject of a detailed interview in Reiki Magazine International (1999). And her work was mentioned in Dog Fancy (2001). She was the subject of a special feature by ACCESS TV/Canadian Learning Television.

Susan has lived her life surrounded by pets: dogs, cats, rabbits, hamsters, turtles, birds, and an earthworm called Arnold. She shares her home in Sherwood Park, Alberta, Canada with her mixed-breed cats, Kahlua, Christmas Blessing, and Kinky, and her retired show dog Crackle (American Champion Braewood Tarnished Brass).

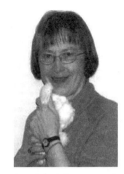

Natalia M. Krawetz

After receiving her doctorate from The City University of New York (environmental psychology, 1978), Natalia Krawetz worked with the private and public sectors on projects related to the social aspects of environmental issues. In 1990 she became owned by a cat who challenged Natalia by contracting unusual maladies that required alternative therapies and behavioral intervention. In response, Natalia enhanced her educational qualifications with a variety of certificates in complementary and alternative modalities: Reiki, Therapeutic Touch and Flower Essence Therapy, as well as in feline behavior. On the advice of her cat, Natalia changed careers in the mid-'90s, establishing a wellness support service for people and cats. She taught in the Holistic Health Practitioner Program at MacEwan College, and offered cat courses for the public at Metro College, and for veterinarians and animal health technologists at The Northern Alberta Institute of Technology and Fairview College.

She served on the Edmonton SPCA Board (1992 - 97), chairing its Pet Population and Planning Committees, and becoming a Vice-President. She was the public member of the Alberta Veterinary Medical Association Task Force that set the provincial guidelines for the practice of holistic veterinary medicine (1998).

Her articles and reports include: "Getting a Handle on Companion Animal Overpopulation," ESPCA Shelter Bulletin, Dec. 1994; "Back in Line: Cats Who Have Chiropractic," Tiger Tribe, Sept./Oct. 1995; "Advances in Pheromontherapy for the Treatment of Urine Marking in Cats," Alberta Association of Aninal Health Technologist's Newsletter, 14 (4), August 1998; and a variety of articles for local pet magazines and newsletters.

She appeared weekly on the national, one-hour television show, HelpTV (ACCESS TV/Canadian Learning Television), responding to callers questions about cats and occasionally hosting short features. In 2002, she participated as the expert resource in the episode on Pain Management, for the television series Healing with Animals.

She retired in 2001. She lives in Edmonton, Alberta, Canada with her husband, Bill MacDonald, and their cat, Precious Greyce.

Other Books Published
by
Ozark Mountain Publishing, Inc.

For more information about any of the above titles, soon to be released
titles, or other items in our catalog, write or visit our website:

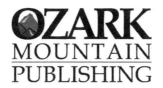

PO Box 754
Huntsville, AR 72740
www.ozarkmt.com
1-800-935-0045/479-738-2348 Wholesale Inquiries Welcome